UNRAVELING DIABETES

A Comprehensive Guide to Understanding and Managing the Condition

By

John E. Ramirez

Author's Disclaimer

The contents of this book are intended for informational purposes only and should not be considered a substitute for professional medical, nutritional, or psychological advice, diagnosis, or treatment. The author is not a medical professional, and the information provided is based on personal research and experience. Readers are encouraged to consult with qualified healthcare professionals for any specific health concerns, conditions, or dietary needs. Any actions or decisions made based on the information in this book are the sole responsibility of the reader.

By reading this book, the reader acknowledges and accepts these disclaimers. It is advised to consult a qualified healthcare professional for any medical, nutritional, or psychological concerns.

TABLE OF CONTENTS

Introduction: The Rise of Diabetes

Diabetes has become a rising health concern in recent years, affecting the lives of millions of people worldwide. Diabetes has progressed from a relatively obscure ailment to a global epidemic affecting individuals of all ages, races, and socioeconomic backgrounds, with worrisome rates of increase. As we watch this historic surge, it is more important than ever to untangle the complexity of diabetes and shine a light on its far-reaching impact on individuals, families, and communities.

"Unraveling Diabetes: A Comprehensive Guide to Understanding and Managing the Condition," chapter by chapter, takes you on a trip through the intricate web of diabetes, beginning with an exploration of its various forms and how they present in different people. We investigate the underlying causes and risk factors, dispelling the mysterious relationship between genetics, lifestyle decisions, and the development of diabetes. With this knowledge, you will be better able to recognize warning signs and take appropriate action to protect your health.

We look at the glycemic index and glycemic load, giving you skills to make informed meal-planning decisions and understand the impact of different food choices on your health. We hope to break down barriers and help you find joy in being active by providing practical advice and guidance.

"Unraveling Diabetes" acknowledges the emotional toll that diabetes may have. Coping with the diagnosis and day-to-day issues can be difficult, but we provide ways to promote mental well-being and resilience.

This thorough guide is designed to provide you with the tools you need to survive despite the obstacles of diabetes. We offer practical advice for everyday life, from traveling with diabetes to managing it at work or school. By the end of this journey, you will be able to take care of your health, make informed decisions, and navigate life with diabetes with confidence.

"Unraveling Diabetes" is more than a book; it is a companion, a source of knowledge, and a ray of hope for anyone seeking to understand the complexity of diabetes and reclaim control of their health. Join us on this life-changing journey as we unravel the keys to understanding and managing diabetes one page at a time.

CHAPTER ONE
Understanding Diabetes

Diabetes is a chronic metabolic illness that affects how our bodies process glucose, which is our cells' principal source of energy. Carbohydrates are broken down into glucose, which enters our circulation when we consume them. In reaction, the pancreas secretes insulin, a hormone that promotes glucose uptake by our cells, allowing them to use it for energy.

Diabetes is a long-term medical illness that affects the body's ability to manage blood sugar levels. It happens when the pancreas does not create enough insulin or when the body does not use the insulin that is produced adequately.

Insulin is a hormone that allows glucose to enter cells and be used as energy, thereby helping to regulate blood sugar (glucose) levels. This process is disrupted in diabetes, resulting in elevated blood sugar levels.

This delicate balance is disrupted in diabetics, resulting in abnormal glucose levels in the bloodstream. Diabetes is classified into two types, the most common of which are Type 1 and Type 2 diabetes.

Managing Diabetes:

Diabetes management focuses on keeping blood glucose levels within a healthy range to avoid complications. Lifestyle changes such as a balanced diet, regular physical activity, and weight management may be part of treatment strategies. Insulin therapy is required for Type 1 diabetes patients, while Type 2 diabetes patients may also require oral medications or other injectable therapies.

Monitoring blood glucose levels is an important part of diabetes management because it allows people to make informed decisions about their diet, medication, and overall health. Regular medical check-ups and screenings for diabetes-related complications are also necessary to detect potential problems early and prevent them from progressing.

Diabetes necessitates a proactive approach to health and a commitment to self-care. Individuals with diabetes can take charge of their health and live fulfilling lives while effectively managing their condition if they understand the condition, its various forms, and the factors that influence it. Furthermore, diabetes education and awareness within the broader community are critical to promoting prevention and supporting those affected by the condition.

Types of Diabetes

Diabetes is classified into several types, each with its own set of characteristics, causes, and management strategies. The main types of diabetes are:

1. Type 1 Diabetes
   Type 1 diabetes, also known as insulin-dependent diabetes or juvenile diabetes, is an autoimmune disease in which the body's immune system attacks and destroys insulin-producing beta cells in the pancreas. As a result, the pancreas produces little to no

insulin, resulting in hyperglycemia. People with Type 1 diabetes require insulin therapy for the rest of their lives in order to control their blood sugar levels and stay alive. Diabetes of this type is typically diagnosed in childhood or adolescence, but it can occur at any age.

2. Type 2 Diabetes
Type 2 diabetes is the most common type of diabetes. It happens when the body becomes resistant to the effects of insulin or produces insufficient insulin to meet

the body's needs. Sedentary behavior, poor diet, obesity, and genetics are all strongly associated with this condition. Type 2 diabetes, unlike Type 1 diabetes, is frequently manageable through lifestyle changes, oral medications, injectable medications, or a combination of these approaches.

3. Gestational Diabetes

Gestational diabetes, a type of diabetes, occurs only during pregnancy. Pregnancy hormone changes can impair insulin sensitivity, resulting in high blood glucose levels. Gestational diabetes usually resolves after childbirth. Women who have had gestational diabetes, on the other hand, are at a higher risk of developing Type 2 diabetes later in life.

4. Prediabetes

Prediabetes is a condition whereby the blood glucose levels are higher than normal but is not higher than the Type 2 diabetes. It is regarded as a red flag, indicating an increased risk of Type 2 diabetes and cardiovascular disease. In many cases, however, lifestyle changes such as adopting a healthy diet and increasing physical activity can prevent or delay the onset of Type 2 diabetes.

Other Types of Diabetes:

Other, less common types of diabetes can be caused by certain medical conditions or medications. Certain medications, such as corticosteroids, can, for example, cause drug-induced diabetes. Other types of diabetes include maturity-onset diabetes of the young (MODY), a genetic form of diabetes that often manifests at a younger age, and secondary diabetes, which develops as a result of another medical condition such as pancreatitis or cystic fibrosis.

Understanding the various types of diabetes is critical for accurate diagnosis, treatment, and management. Each type necessitates a customized approach to ensure that individuals receive the care and support they require to maintain their health and well-being.

Regular medical exams and screenings are essential for detecting diabetes early and implementing effective diabetes management strategies. We can work toward better diabetes prevention, management, and support by raising awareness and understanding the complexities of the disease.

Causes and Risk Factors

Diabetes develops as a result of a combination of genetic, lifestyle, and environmental factors.

Understanding the causes and risk factors for diabetes can assist individuals and healthcare professionals in identifying those at higher risk and implementing preventive or early intervention measures. Here are some of the major causes and risk factors for diabetes:

1. Genetics: Diabetes in the family can increase the risk of developing the condition. Certain genes are linked to an increased susceptibility to Type 1 and Type 2 diabetes, but having these genes does

not guarantee that you will get the disease.

2. Obesity: Being overweight is one of the major reasons for developing Type 2 diabetes. Excess body fat, particularly around the abdomen, can lead to insulin resistance, a condition in which the cells of the body do not respond effectively to insulin.

3. Lack of physical activity: Sedentary lifestyles and a lack of regular physical activity can both contribute to the development of Type 2 diabetes. Exercise improves

insulin utilization and can prevent or postpone the onset of diabetes.

4. Unhealthy Diet: A diet high in processed foods, sugary beverages, and unhealthy fats can contribute to insulin resistance and increase the risk of Type 2 diabetes. Furthermore, diets low in fiber and nutrient-rich foods can have a negative impact on blood glucose control.

5. Age: The risk of developing diabetes rises with age, especially in Type 2 diabetes. This is due in part to aging-

related factors such as decreased physical activity and changes in body composition.

6. Ethnicity: Some ethnic groups are more likely than others to develop diabetes. Individuals of African, Hispanic, Asian, or Native American descent, for example, have a higher risk of Type 2 diabetes.

7. Gestational Diabetes History: Women who have had gestational diabetes during their pregnancy are more

likely to develop Type 2 diabetes later in life.

8. Polycystic Ovary Syndrome (PCOS): Women who have PCOS, a hormonal disorder that can cause irregular menstrual cycles and infertility, are more likely to develop insulin resistance and Type 2 diabetes.

9. High Blood Pressure: Hypertension, also known as high blood pressure, is a risk factor for Type 2 diabetes and can exacerbate complications in diabetics.

10.   High Cholesterol and Triglyceride Levels: In diabetics, abnormal lipid levels in the blood can increase the risk of cardiovascular complications.

11.   History of Cardiovascular Disease: Individuals with a family history of heart disease or stroke are at a higher risk of developing Type 2 diabetes.

12.   Sleep Disorders: Because of their impact on insulin sensitivity, conditions such as sleep apnea have

been linked to an increased risk of Type 2 diabetes.

While some diabetes risk factors, such as age and family history, cannot be changed, others, such as weight, physical activity, and diet, can be managed through lifestyle changes. Regular check-ups, early detection, and proactive management can all help to lessen the impact of diabetes and its complications. Identifying and addressing risk factors early on can empower people to take control of their health and make informed decisions to effectively prevent or manage diabetes.

Signs and Symptoms

Diabetes signs and symptoms vary depending on the type of diabetes and the individual. It is critical to be aware of these symptoms because early detection and treatment are critical for effectively managing the condition. The following are the most common signs and symptoms of Type 1 and Type 2 diabetes:

Common Diabetes Signs and Symptoms:

1. Frequent Urination (Polyuria): Diabetics may experience frequent urination, particularly at night. This happens because the kidneys work to remove excess glucose from the bloodstream by excreting it in the urine.

2. Polydipsia (Increased Thirst): Frequent urination can cause dehydration, resulting in increased thirst as the body

attempts to replenish lost fluids.

3. Unexplained Weight Loss: Individuals with Type 1 diabetes may experience unexplained weight loss due to the body's inability to use glucose for energy, resulting in the breakdown of fat and muscle tissues.

4. Fatigue and Weakness: In both Type 1 and Type 2 diabetes, the cells of the body may not receive enough glucose for energy, resulting in fatigue and weakness.

5. Blurry Vision: High blood glucose levels can alter the shape of the eye's lens, resulting in temporary blurry vision.

6. Slow Healing of Wounds: Diabetes can impair the body's ability to heal wounds, resulting in slow healing and an increased risk of infection.

7. Frequent Infections: Because high blood glucose levels weaken the immune system, diabetics are more prone to infections, particularly in the urinary tract, skin, and gums.

8. Tingling or Numbness in Hands and Feet: High blood glucose levels for an extended period of time can damage nerves, resulting in peripheral neuropathy, which is characterized by tingling, numbness, or pain in the hands and feet.

Additional Signs of Type 1 Diabetes:

1. Extreme Hunger (Polyphagia): The cells in the body do not receive enough glucose for energy, resulting

in increased hunger and food intake.

2. Ketones in Urine: When the body is unable to utilize glucose for energy, it begins to break down fat for energy, which results in the formation of ketones. Ketone levels in the urine can be elevated, which may indicate diabetic ketoacidosis, a serious complication of Type 1 diabetes.

It's important to remember that some people may have moderate or atypical symptoms, while others may not have any symptoms at all, especially in the early stages of Type 2 diabetes. Regular health examinations and blood glucose testing are critical for the early detection and management of diabetes.

If you or someone you know has any of these symptoms or feels they may have diabetes, seek medical help immediately for the correct diagnosis and treatment. Early detection and care can help prevent complications and enhance the quality of life for people with diabetes.

Diagnosing Diabetes

Diabetes is diagnosed by analyzing an individual's blood glucose levels and other clinical signs to determine if they have the disease. Diabetes can lead to serious problems if left untreated, thus early identification is critical for establishing proper treatment and management methods. A variety of tests are used to diagnose diabetes and establish its type. The following are the most common diagnostic criteria:

1. FPG (Fasting Plasma Glucose) Test: This test

measures blood glucose levels following at least an 8-hour overnight fast. Before breakfast, a blood sample is collected. Diabetes is commonly diagnosed when the fasting plasma glucose level is 126 milligrams per deciliter (mg/dL) or greater on two separate occasions.

2. Oral Glucose Tolerance Test (OGTT): This test measures a person's blood glucose levels following an overnight fast. They are then asked to drink a glucose-rich solution, after which blood samples are

obtained at regular intervals for the next two hours. If the blood glucose level is 200 mg/dL or greater two hours after drinking the solution, diabetes is verified.

3. Hemoglobin A1c(HbA1c) Test: The hemoglobin A1c (HbA1c) test offers an average of a person's blood glucose levels over the previous two to three months. It calculates the percentage of hemoglobin in the blood that is glucose-bound. Diabetes is diagnosed when the HbA1c level is 6.5% or greater.

4. Random Plasma Glucose Test: In circumstances where diabetes symptoms are severe, a random blood glucose test without fasting may be conducted. A random plasma glucose level of 200 mg/dL or greater, together with typical diabetic symptoms (excessive thirst, frequent urination, unexplained weight loss), can confirm a diabetes diagnosis.

It is critical to emphasize that a diabetes diagnosis should not rely solely on a single test result.

Multiple tests are usually required to confirm the diagnosis and rule out other possible reasons for high blood glucose levels.

For determining the various forms of diabetes:

Type 1 diabetes is frequently diagnosed based on symptoms and a high blood glucose level. Autoantibodies, which are antibodies that attack the body's own tissues, can also assist distinguish Type 1 diabetes from Type 2 diabetes.

Type 2 Diabetes: The diagnostic criteria for Type 2 diabetes are the same as those for Type 1 diabetes. In order to distinguish between Type 1 and Type 2 diabetes, healthcare providers may also consider the patient's age, body weight, and family history.

Gestational Diabetes: Gestational diabetes is diagnosed with an OGTT, which is usually performed between 24 and 28 weeks of pregnancy. At that time, a high blood glucose level implies gestational diabetes.

Diagnosis of diabetes is not only necessary for controlling the condition but also for implementing preventative interventions and lifestyle adjustments for those at risk. Regular check-ups and screenings are critical for early identification and timely intervention, which contributes to improved health outcomes and a higher quality of life for diabetics.

CHAPTER TWO
Demystifying Blood Glucose

Blood glucose, otherwise called blood sugar, is a significant part of our body's energy guideline. It alludes to the centralization of glucose (a sort of sugar) present in our circulatory system at some random time. Glucose is the essential wellspring of energy for our cells, and keeping up with the right degree of blood glucose is fundamental for by and large wellbeing and prosperity.

The amount of sugar (glucose) in the bloodstream is measured as blood glucose. It is a necessary component of the body's energy synthesis and is regulated by the pancreatic hormone insulin.

Carbohydrates are broken down into glucose and released into the bloodstream when we eat them. This raises blood glucose levels. In reaction, the pancreas secretes insulin to aid in the transport of glucose from the bloodstream into cells, where it can be used for energy.

It is critical for overall health to keep blood glucose levels steady. Blood glucose levels that are too high or too low might cause a variety of health concerns.

Hyperglycemia, or high blood glucose levels, can develop in diabetics or in persons who have consumed a substantial amount of carbohydrates. Increased thirst, frequent urination, weariness, and blurred vision are all symptoms of high blood glucose. Long-term high blood glucose levels can cause kidney damage, neurological damage, and other issues and cardiovascular problems.

Hypoglycemia, or low blood glucose levels, can induce symptoms such as shakiness, dizziness, sweating, and confusion. Diabetes patients who use insulin or other diabetes treatments may experience hypoglycemia. It can also happen to those who haven't eaten in a long time or who have done a lot of physical exercise without eating enough carbohydrates.

Individuals with diabetes must frequently test their blood glucose levels in order to manage their blood glucose levels. A glucometer, a tiny instrument that monitors glucose levels in a drop of blood collected from a finger prick, is commonly used for this. The findings can assist individuals in making informed decisions about nutrition, medication, and exercise in order to maintain ideal blood glucose levels.

Aside from monitoring, lifestyle variables such as a nutritious diet, frequent physical activity, and maintaining a healthy weight can all help to manage blood glucose levels. Eating a well-balanced diet high in fiber and low in refined sugars can help manage blood glucose levels. Physical activity, particularly aerobic exercise, can enhance insulin sensitivity and aid with blood glucose control.

Understanding blood glucose and its management is critical for diabetics as well as healthcare professionals who diagnose and manage the disease. Effective blood glucose management can help diabetics live healthy and productive lives while lowering the risk of diabetes-related complications.

The Role of Insulin

Insulin is a hormone generated by the pancreas, primarily by beta cells in the Langerhans islets. Its principal function is to control the levels of glucose in the bloodstream. Carbohydrates are broken down into glucose and released into the bloodstream when we eat them. This causes blood glucose levels to rise, causing the pancreas to release insulin.

Insulin works by telling various cells in the body to absorb glucose from the bloodstream, primarily muscle, fat, and liver cells. Insulin increases glucose uptake and conversion into glycogen, a glucose storage form, in muscle cells. Insulin stimulates the storage of glucose as triglycerides in fat cells, resulting in fat gain.

Insulin slows the release of glucose from glycogen stores and stimulates its conversion into glycogen for storage in the liver.

In addition to regulating glucose levels, insulin is involved in protein synthesis and fat metabolism. It promotes protein synthesis and muscle growth by increasing the absorption of amino acids by cells. Insulin also prevents fat breakdown and promotes fat accumulation in adipose tissue.

Insulin synthesis or function is compromised in diabetics, resulting in poor blood glucose regulation. Type 1 diabetes is an autoimmune disease in which the body's immune system targets and destroys beta cells in the pancreas, resulting in little or no insulin production. Individuals with type 1 diabetes must therefore rely on external insulin therapy.

Type 2 diabetes, on the other hand, is characterized by insulin resistance, in which the body's cells become less receptive to the actions of insulin. This can result in inadequate glucose absorption and high blood glucose levels. Over time, the pancreas may also fail to generate enough insulin to overcome insulin resistance, aggravating the illness.

Insulin therapy is a frequent treatment for both type 1 and type 2 diabetes. Individuals with type 1 diabetes must administer insulin injections or utilize an insulin pump to control their blood glucose levels. Insulin therapy is typically administered in type 2 diabetes when other drugs and lifestyle changes are no longer sufficient to control blood glucose levels.

Overall, insulin regulates blood glucose levels, promotes glucose uptake into cells, and maintains overall metabolic balance. Understanding the role of insulin in diabetes management and maintaining good blood glucose control is critical.

Self-Testing and Glucose Monitoring

Individuals with diabetes must use glucose monitoring and self-testing to appropriately manage their blood glucose levels. It entails measuring blood glucose levels on a regular basis with a glucose meter or continuous glucose monitoring system

(CGM). This enables people to make educated decisions about their nutrition, medications, and lifestyle choices in order to maintain optimal blood glucose control.

Traditional Glucose Monitoring:

1. Glucometers: Glucometers are handheld devices that use a little drop of blood acquired by a finger prick to measure blood glucose levels. Within seconds, the meter reads the glucose level and displays it on a screen. Individuals can then use this

data to alter their insulin dosage or take other necessary actions to keep their blood glucose levels within desired ranges.

2. Test Strips: Glucometers are used in combination with test strips. They are placed in the meter, and a drop of blood is added to the measurement strip. Based on the glucose level in the blood sample, the glucose meter then produces a readout.

Continuous Glucose Monitoring (CGM)

1. CGM Systems: Throughout the day, CGM systems give continuous, real-time glucose measurements. Wearing a small sensor implanted under the skin, generally on the abdomen or arm, is required. The sensor detects glucose levels in the interstitial fluid and wirelessly transfers the information to a receiver or smartphone. Users can access their glucose levels at any

moment, as well as track trends and patterns over time.

2. Alerts and Alarms: CGM systems can be designed to generate alerts and alarms when glucose levels are abnormally high or low. This can assist folks in taking prompt action to avoid issues.

The Advantages of Glucose Monitoring and Self-Testing:

1. Individualized Management: Regular glucose monitoring enables people to learn how their bodies react to various diets, exercise, medications,

and daily activities. This aids in the development of a tailored management strategy for maintaining stable blood glucose levels.

2. Treatment Modification: By monitoring blood glucose levels, people can alter their insulin dosage or take the right drugs based on their results. It aids in tighter glucose control and lowers the risk of diabetes-related complications.

3. Detection of Hypoglycemia and Hyperglycemia: Glucose monitoring aids in the

identification of low blood sugar (hypoglycemia) and high blood sugar (hyperglycemia) events. This enables people to take quick action, such as eating carbohydrate-rich foods to address hypoglycemia or modifying medication to correct hyperglycemia.

4. Trend Analysis: Blood glucose levels should be monitored and tracked on a regular basis to discover trends and patterns. This enables people to make informed diabetes

management decisions, such as changing their diet, exercise routine, or medication regimen.

5. Self-Care and Empowerment: Glucose monitoring puts people in charge of their diabetes management. It gives individuals the ability to actively participate in their own care and make lifestyle decisions that encourage optimal blood glucose management.

It is critical to adhere to the frequency and timing of glucose monitoring as prescribed by healthcare professionals.

Interpreting Blood Glucose Results

Individuals with diabetes and healthcare professionals involved in maintaining and treating the condition must be able to interpret blood glucose data. Understanding the relevance of blood glucose levels can aid in the direction of treatment decisions and lifestyle changes to maintain optimal blood glucose management. Here are some important considerations to keep in mind while evaluating blood glucose results:

1. Blood Glucose Target Range: There are typically recommended blood glucose target ranges, which may vary depending on factors such as age, type of diabetes, and overall health. Blood glucose levels should typically be between 80-130 mg/dL before meals (preprandial), and less than 180 mg/dL 1-2 hours after meals (postprandial).

2. Hypoglycemia occurs when blood glucose levels fall below the normal range (typically less than 70 mg/dL or 3.9 mmol/L). Shaking, sweating, disorientation, and weakness are all possible symptoms. To treat hypoglycemia, take immediate action, such as taking a fast-acting source of glucose, such as fruit juice or glucose pills.

3. Hyperglycemia: Hyperglycemia is defined as elevated blood glucose levels that are typically over the

target range. Hyperglycemia can cause symptoms such as increased thirst, frequent urination, lethargy, and impaired vision, depending on the degree. Long-term hyperglycemia can lead to issues such as kidney disease, nerve damage, and cardiovascular disease. To lower blood glucose levels and avoid problems, medication, food, and lifestyle changes may be required.

4. Trend Analysis: It is critical to examine not only

individual blood glucose levels but also trends over time. Monitoring patterns in blood glucose levels can aid in the identification of probable triggers or variables influencing swings. For example, if persistently higher readings occur after specific meals or at specified times of day, meal planning, medication timing, or physical activity may need to be adjusted.

5. Individual Variations: Every person's blood glucose reaction is unique. Some

people may have better control with narrower target ranges, whereas others may have more flexible target ranges. Working together with healthcare specialists to develop individualized target ranges based on individual circumstances and health goals is critical.

Remember that analyzing blood glucose levels should be done in cooperation with healthcare specialists who can provide tailored advice and recommendations. Regular communication and data exchange about blood glucose levels enables appropriate adjustments to treatment programs and lifestyle changes to achieve optimal blood glucose control and overall diabetes care.

CHAPTER THREE
Nutrition and Diet Management

Nutrition and food management are important parts of diabetes care because they help manage blood glucose levels, promote general health, and prevent diabetes-related complications. A well-balanced and well-planned diet can help diabetics improve their blood sugar management, maintain a healthy weight, and lower their risk of cardiovascular disease. Here are some basic nutritional and diet management guidelines for diabetics:

1. Carbohydrate Sensitivity: Carbohydrates have a direct impact on blood glucose levels, thus it's critical to watch your carbohydrate consumption. Carbohydrates can be found in grains, fruits & vegetables, dairy products, and sweets.

2. Carbohydrates Counting or Budgeting: Carbohydrates can help diabetics maintain their blood glucose levels by matching insulin dosages or

medications to the amount of carbohydrates taken in meals and snacks.

3. Choose Nutrient-Dense Whole Foods: Choose nutrient-dense whole foods that are high in vitamins, minerals, and fiber. Include entire grains, fruits and vegetables, lean proteins, and healthy fats in your diet. These foods have a slower effect on blood glucose levels and make you feel full and invigorated.

4. Balanced Meals: Aim for meals that are well-balanced

in terms of carbohydrates, proteins, and healthy fats. A balanced plate should include half of non-starchy vegetables, one-quarter of lean protein, and one-quarter of whole grains or other nutritious carbohydrates.

5. Portion Management: To avoid overeating and efficiently manage blood glucose levels, pay proper attention to portion sizes. To avoid consuming too many calories, use smaller dishes and pay attention to serving sizes.

6. Limit Added Sugars and Processed Carbohydrates: Limit your intake of sugary snacks, sodas, and baked goods, which are high in added sugars and processed carbohydrates. These can cause blood glucose increase and contribute to weight gain.

7. Healthy Fats: Include avocados, almonds, seeds, and olive oil in your diet as sources of healthy fats. These fats can aid insulin sensitivity and heart health.

8. Keep an eye on your sodium intake: Consuming too much

sodium (salt) can have a negative impact on blood pressure and cardiovascular health. Choose low-sodium choices and flavor foods with herbs and spices rather than salt.

9. Stay Hydrated: To stay hydrated, drink plenty of water throughout the day. Sugary beverages and fruit juices should be avoided because they can elevate blood glucose levels.

10.   Meal Timing: Eating at regular intervals can help manage blood glucose levels

and promote insulin sensitivity. Try to consume meals and snacks at consistent times throughout the day.

11.   Individualized Approach: Because nutritional requirements differ from person to person, it is critical to take an individualized approach to diet management. Work with a licensed dietitian or diabetes educator to create a personalized meal plan that fits your tastes, lifestyle, and health objectives.

Individuals with diabetes can effectively manage their disease and enhance their overall well-being by making smart food choices, exercising portion control, and keeping physically active. Regular blood glucose monitoring, together with a balanced diet and a healthy lifestyle, can help people with diabetes live full and active lives while reducing the risk of diabetes-related complications.

Carbohydrates, Proteins, and Fats: Balancing Macronutrients

Balancing macronutrients (carbohydrates, proteins, and fats) is an important aspect of nutrition and diet management, especially for diabetics. Each macronutrient performs a different role in the body and has a varied effect on blood glucose levels. A well-balanced diet with the proper amounts of these nutrients can help regulate blood glucose, maintain general health, and effectively manage weight. The following is a breakdown of each macronutrient and its significance in a healthy diet:

1. Carbohydrates:
   Carbohydrates are the body's major source of energy, and they have the greatest influence on blood glucose levels. Carbohydrates are converted into glucose, which enters the bloodstream and elevates blood sugar levels. Individuals with diabetes must carefully monitor their carbohydrate consumption to minimize blood glucose rises.

a. Types of Carbohydrates
There are simple and complex carbohydrates

- Simple Carbohydrates Sugars, candies, baked goods, and sweetened beverages are examples of simple carbohydrates. They digest quickly and can result in rapid spikes in blood glucose levels.
- Complex Carbohydrates

Whole grains, legumes, fruits, and vegetables are all high sources of complex carbohydrates. Complex carbohydrates digest at a slower rate, resulting in a more steady and persistent release of glucose into the bloodstream.

b. Balancing Carbohydrate: It is critical for diabetics to distribute carbohydrate intake throughout the day, focusing on nutrient-dense, complex carbs that are high in fiber. Carbohydrate counting or budgeting can assist in efficiently managing blood glucose levels.

2. Proteins:
Proteins are required for the formation and repair of tissues, enzymes, hormones, and immunological function. Proteins, unlike carbohydrates, have little effect on blood glucose

levels. Excess protein ingestion, on the other hand, can be turned into glucose via a process known as gluconeogenesis.

a. Protein Sources: Lean meats, poultry, fish, eggs, tofu, lentils, and low-fat dairy products are all good sources of protein. Plant-based proteins such as beans, lentils, and quinoa are good vegetarian and vegan options.

b. Balancing Protein: Include a lean protein

source in each meal to increase satiety and support muscle maintenance and repair. Balanced meals with protein, carbohydrates, and healthy fats can help keep blood glucose levels stable.

3. Fats:

Fats are necessary for several biological activities, including nutrient absorption, hormone generation, and organ insulation. Fats have little direct effect on blood glucose levels, but they are high in calories and can influence overall calorie consumption and weight management.

a. Types of Fats: There are healthy or unhealthy fats:

- Healthy Fats: Monounsaturated and polyunsaturated fats, found in olive oil, avocados, almonds, and seeds, are heart-healthy and can increase insulin sensitivity.

- Unhealthy Fats: Saturated and trans fats, which can be found in processed meals, fried foods, and fatty meats, should be avoided since they can elevate cholesterol levels and increase the risk of heart disease.

b. Balancing Fat: Incorporate healthy fats into your diet in moderation. Incorporate monounsaturated and polyunsaturated fats into your diet instead of saturated and trans fats.

Focus on full, nutrient-dense foods and keep portion sizes in mind to attain a well-balanced diet. To encourage stable blood glucose levels and overall health, balance your meals by including a variety of carbohydrates, proteins, and healthy fats. Working with a registered dietitian or diabetes educator can help you establish a meal plan that is tailored to your specific health goals and needs. Regular blood glucose monitoring and making informed food choices can lead to better diabetes management and overall well-being.

Glycemic Index and Glycemic Load

The Glycemic Index (GI) and Glycemic Load (GL) are two key concepts in understanding how carbohydrates in foods affect blood glucose levels. They are useful tools for diabetics and others attempting to efficiently regulate their blood sugar levels. Understanding the GI and GL of foods will help you make more informed dietary choices and improve your blood glucose control.

GI (Glycemic Index):

The Glycemic Index is a numerical scale that classifies carbohydrates in foods according to how rapidly and significantly they elevate blood glucose levels when compared to pure glucose (a reference value of 100). Foods with a high GI digest quickly and induce a spike in blood sugar. Those with a low GI digest more slowly, resulting in a gradual rise in blood glucose.

GI Categories:

Low GI: 55 or less

GI Medium: 56-69

High GI: 70 or higher

Example: White bread has a high GI (about 70-85), which means it induces a quick surge in blood glucose when consumed. Whole grains, on the other hand, have a lower GI (approximately 25-55), resulting in a slower rise in blood sugar.

GL (Glycemic Load):

The Glycemic Load considers both the GI and the actual amount of carbohydrates in a portion of food, whereas the GI ranks meals primarily on their immediate influence on blood glucose levels. The GL is a more practical assessment of how a company operates.

Calculating GL

GL is computed using the following formula: GL = (GI x Carbohydrate content in grams per serving) / 100.

Example: Watermelon has a high GI (about 72) yet has a low carbohydrate content per serving.

As a result, its GL is moderate: GL = (72 x 6g carbs) / 100 = 4.32.

A low-GI food may have a high GL if it includes a lot of carbs per serving.

How to Use GI and GL to Manage Diabetes

Low-GI meals digest more slowly, resulting in a more gradual rise in blood glucose levels. These foods are often healthier choices for people with diabetes since they help keep blood sugar levels constant.

High-GI foods can trigger blood glucose rises, making them less desirable choices, especially when consumed alone. When coupled with other foods, particularly ones that slow digestion (such as proteins or healthy fats), the overall influence on blood sugar levels may be mitigated.

Considering both GI and GL can help diabetics make better meal choices. To manage the overall Glycemic Load of a meal, choose low-GI items and watch portion amounts.

While GI and GL are useful tools, it's important to note that everyone's reactions to food differ. Individual metabolism, total food composition, and other nutrients in a meal can all have an impact on blood glucose levels. As a result, it's recommended to use GI and GL as part of a comprehensive, tailored diabetes treatment strategy overseen by a healthcare expert or registered dietitian.

Meal Planning and Portion Control

When it comes to diabetes management, meal planning, and portion control are essential. They can help control blood sugar levels and maintain a healthy diet. Here are some diabetes-specific meal planning and portion control tips:

1. Space meals evenly throughout the day: To assist maintain stable blood sugar levels, aim for regular meals and snacks spaced regularly throughout the day. Do not

skip meals or fast for an extended period.

2. Include a macronutrient balance: Each meal should have a combination of carbohydrates, proteins, and healthy fats. This aids in blood sugar regulation and gives long-lasting energy.

3. Carbohydrate counting: Learn to count carbohydrates in order to maintain blood sugar levels accurately. Consult a qualified dietitian or a healthcare expert to assess your carbohydrate requirements and how to

incorporate them into your diet. Remember to prioritize complex carbohydrates like whole grains, legumes, and veggies above simple carbohydrates like sugar.

4. Portion control: Pay attention to portion proportions to avoid overeating and to keep calorie consumption under control. To visually measure portion sizes, use smaller plates and measuring cups. To determine recommended portion sizes for your unique needs, speak with a licensed nutritionist.

5. Choose foods with a low glycemic index (GI): To help reduce blood sugar levels, choose foods with a low GI. Non-starchy veggies, whole grains, and legumes are examples. High-GI foods, such as refined grains, sugary snacks, and sugary beverages, should be avoided or limited.

6. Choose lean protein sources, such as skinless fowl, fish, tofu, lentils, and low-fat dairy products. Protein regulates blood sugar levels and keeps you satisfied.

7. Watch your fat intake: Aim for healthy fats such as avocados, nuts, seeds, and olive oil. Because fats are high in calories, moderation is essential. Limit your intake of saturated and trans fats, which can be found in fried foods, fatty meats, full-fat dairy products, and processed snacks.

8. Fiber-rich foods: Eat lots of fiber-rich foods such as fruits, vegetables, whole grains, and legumes. Fiber slows carbohydrate

absorption and helps manage blood sugar levels.

9. Cook at home: Cooking at home gives you control over the ingredients and portion proportions. It can also be less expensive and healthier than dining out or relying on processed foods.

10. Consult a certified dietitian: Speak with a registered dietitian who specializes in diabetes to develop a tailored food plan that meets your needs, lifestyle, and goals. They may advise you on meal

planning and quantity control, as well as provide continuous help in controlling your diabetes via nutrition.

The Impacts of Sugar and Artificial Sweeteners

Sugars and artificial sweeteners can also have serious health consequences, especially for people with diabetes or those trying to maintain stable blood glucose levels and overall well-being. Understanding the impacts of sugars and artificial sweeteners can help people make more informed dietary decisions. The following examines each of them:

Sugar's Influence

1. Glucose Levels in the Blood: Sugary foods, especially those with added sugars, can cause fast rises in blood glucose levels. Individuals with diabetes may find it difficult to manage these unexpected rises since they necessitate appropriate insulin doses or prescription modifications.

2. Weight Control: Sugary foods are generally high in

calories but low in nutritious value. Sugary meals and beverages can cause weight gain or difficulties regulating weight, which can impair blood glucose regulation and increase the risk of numerous health problems.

3. Insulin Resistance: A high-sugar diet has been linked to a higher risk of insulin resistance, a condition in which cells become less receptive to insulin, resulting in higher blood glucose levels.

Sugary meals and beverages contribute to tooth decay and cavities, which can be detrimental to general oral health.

The Effect of Artificial Sweeteners:

1. Blood Glucose Level: Artificial sweeteners are non-caloric or low-caloric sugar alternatives that do not normally elevate blood glucose levels. They can be advantageous to diabetics since they give sweetness without influencing blood sugar levels. Individuals'

reactions to artificial sweeteners, on the other hand, can differ.

2. Weight Control: Artificial sweeteners are frequently employed as a sugar substitute in "diet" or "low-calorie" products because they give sweetness without the extra calories of sugar. While some studies suggest that artificial sweeteners may help with weight loss by lowering overall calorie intake, other research has raised problems, such as

increased cravings for sweet foods.

3. Taste Perception: Some people may discover that taking artificial sweeteners on a regular basis changes their taste preferences, causing them to seek sweeter foods and beverages. This can result in a preference for excessively sweetened foods and a dislike for naturally sweet foods such as fruits.

4. Digestive Health: Consuming significant doses of artificial sweeteners may cause stomach discomfort or other

adverse effects in some people.

Overall Suggestions:

1. Balance and moderation: Moderation is essential whether you use sugar or artificial sweeteners. Reducing overall sugar consumption benefits general health, including improved blood glucose control.

2. Examine the Labels: Be on the lookout for hidden sugars in packaged and processed foods. Read nutrition labels and ingredient lists to

discover goods that include added sugars or artificial sweeteners.

3. Emphasis on Whole Foods: When feasible, choose whole, natural foods and beverages over overly processed or sweetened goods.

4. Personalized Approach: Individuals have varying reactions to glucose and artificial sweeteners. Some people may tolerate tiny amounts of natural sugar better, whilst others may find artificial sweeteners useful in controlling blood glucose

levels. It's critical to figure out what works best for you and your specific health demands.

5. Collaboration with a Healthcare Professional: Consult a trained dietician or healthcare practitioner if you have diabetes or other specific health concerns to build a customized dietary plan that meets your health goals and objectives. They can advise you on how to successfully manage sugars and artificial sweeteners in your diet.

Mindful Eating for Diabetes

For those with diabetes, mindful eating can help them manage their illness and improve their relationship with food. Below are some suggestions for mindful eating:

1. Take your time: Eat your meals slowly and mindfully. Carefully chew your food and savor each bite. This allows you to be more aware of your body's hunger and fullness signals.

2. Pay attention to hunger and fullness cues: Assess your

hunger level before eating. Eat when you're physically hungry and stop when you're pleasantly content, not overstuffed. Avoid overeating by paying attention to sensations of hunger and fullness.

3. Pay attention to the current moment: When eating, pay attention to the sensory sensation of the meal. Pay attention to the textures, flavors, and scents. This allows you to truly taste and appreciate your meal and avoids mindless munching.

4. Use all of your senses while eating: Use all of your senses while eating. Enjoy the colors, fragrances, textures, and flavors of your cuisine. This contributes to a more gratifying and delightful dining experience.

5. Pay attention to your body: Be aware of how different foods affect your body. Take note of how particular foods affect your blood sugar levels. Keep a food diary to document your eating habits and how they affect your glucose levels. This will help

you make decisions properly in the future.

6. Practice portion control: Pay attention to portion proportions and feed yourself enough amounts of food. Use smaller dishes and bowls to visibly manage portion sizes.

7. Avoid distractions: Avoid using electronic gadgets or watching television during eating. Concentrate on the act of eating and the sensation of fueling your body.

8. Choose nutrient-dense foods: Make entire, nutrient-dense foods a priority in your

meals. Vegetables, fruits, whole grains, lean meats, and healthy fats are all examples of nutrient-dense foods. These foods supply necessary nutrients and aid with blood sugar regulation.

9. Seek help: Seek advice from a licensed dietitian or diabetic educator who can provide advice on mindful eating and help personalize an eating plan to your specific requirements and goals.

To practice mindful eating, you need time and patience. In implementing mindful eating habits into your routine, be kind to yourself and strive for progress rather than perfection.

CHAPTER FOUR
Exercise and Physical Activity

Exercise and physical exercise are critical in diabetes management. Regular physical activity can help regulate blood sugar levels, enhance insulin sensitivity, and lower the risk of diabetes complications.

When combining exercise and physical activity into a diabetes care strategy, keep the following considerations in mind:

1. Consult with a healthcare professional: It is critical to consult with your healthcare team before beginning an exercise program. They can advise you on the best workouts for your specific needs, as well as any warnings or changes that may be required.

2. Select a range of exercises: Include a variety of aerobic exercises (such as brisk walking, cycling, or swimming), strength training exercises (such as lifting weights or using resistance

bands), and flexibility exercises (such as stretching or yoga) into your exercise routine. This variety aids in the improvement of cardiovascular health, strength, and flexibility.

3. Strive for consistency: Consistent physical activity is essential for diabetes treatment. Go for at least 150 minutes of moderate physical activity three times every week. Increase the duration or intensity of your activity if time allows for further benefits.

4. Check blood sugar levels: Check your blood glucose levels before, during, and after exercise on a regular basis. This will allow you to better understand how your body reacts to various activities and modify your carbohydrate intake or insulin dosage accordingly. If your blood sugar levels are too high or too low before exercising, you may need to postpone or adjust your activity.

5. Take into account timing: Pay attention to when you

exercise in connection to meals and insulin injections. Exercise after a meal may be effective in preventing hypoglycemia (low blood sugar) or adjusting insulin doses if necessary.

6. Stay hydrated: To stay hydrated, drink plenty of water before, during, and after exercise. Avoid sugary sports drinks in favor of water or low-calorie beverages.

7. Be prepared: Always keep a source of quick-acting carbs on hand, such as glucose

tablets or a small snack, in case of a hypoglycemic incident while exercising.

8. Check your feet regularly: If you have diabetes-related nerve loss (neuropathy), it is critical to evaluate your feet for any signs of injury or blisters. Wear appropriate footwear to safeguard your feet when exercising.

9. Pay attention to your body: If you experience any pain, dizziness, shortness of breath, or other strange symptoms while exercising, stop and get medical attention.

When it comes to adding exercise and physical activity to your diabetes treatment plan, remember that consistency is crucial. Regular blood sugar monitoring and collaboration with your healthcare team will assist ensure that exercise is both safe and effective for you.

Benefits of Exercise for Diabetes

Exercise has several benefits for people with diabetes, making it an important part of diabetes care and overall well-being. Regular physical activity can improve many aspects of diabetes management, including blood glucose control and cardiovascular health. Here are some of the primary advantages of exercising for people with diabetes:

1. Improved Blood Glucose Control: Exercise helps raise insulin sensitivity, allowing the body to utilize insulin more effectively to transfer glucose into cells for energy. This improves blood glucose control and eliminates the

need for extra diabetes medicines or insulin.

2. Reduced Insulin Resistance: Physical activity can help lower insulin resistance, a condition in which the body's cells do not respond adequately to insulin. Reduced insulin resistance improves blood glucose control and lowers the chance of developing Type 2 diabetes.

3. Weight Management: Regular exercise helps with weight loss or maintenance, which is especially important

for people with Type 2 diabetes or who are overweight or obese. Keeping a healthy weight can help with insulin sensitivity and blood glucose control.

4. Lower Cardiovascular Risk: Exercise benefits heart health by lowering blood pressure, increasing cholesterol levels, and boosting circulation. Diabetes complications such as cardiovascular disease are frequent, and regular exercise might help minimize this risk.

5. Stress Reduction: Physical activity is an effective stress reliever and promoter of mental well-being. Individuals with diabetes must manage stress because stress hormones can alter blood glucose levels.

6. Increased Energy Levels: Regular exercise can lead to increased energy levels and overall enhanced physical fitness, making it easier for people to engage in daily activities.

7. Better Sleep: It has been demonstrated that exercise

improves sleep quality, which is critical for general health and diabetes management.

8. Enhance Mood and Mental Health: Endorphins, or "feel-good" hormones, are released during exercise, which can boost mood and lessen feelings of anxiety and sadness, which are common in diabetics.

9. Improved Blood Pressure: Exercise helps to manage blood pressure, which is essential for preventing diabetes-related

complications such as renal disease and cardiovascular problems.

10.   Blood Lipid Management: Physical activity can improve lipid profiles by increasing HDL (good cholesterol) levels and decreasing LDL (bad cholesterol), encouraging better heart health.

11.   Increased Muscle Mass: Strength training activities assist build muscular mass, which can improve overall metabolism and glucose utilization.

12.   Type 2 Diabetes Risk is Reduced: Regular exercise is critical in preventing Type 2 diabetes, especially for people who are at high risk due to family history, being overweight, or leading a sedentary lifestyle.

13.   Social Interaction: Group exercises or physical activities can provide opportunities for social connection and support, building a sense of community and incentive to keep active.

Individuals with diabetes should strive for a combination of aerobic workouts (e.g., walking, running, swimming, cycling) and strength training activities at least three to five times per week to enjoy these benefits. Before beginning an exercise plan, always speak with a healthcare practitioner, especially if you have any pre-existing health concerns or diabetes complications. Individuals can enhance their blood glucose control, overall health, and quality of life by adding regular physical activity to a complete diabetes treatment plan.

Designing an Exercise Routine for Diabetes

Individual fitness levels, interests, and any current health issues should all be considered while developing an exercise plan for diabetes. Here are some tips to help you design an appropriate fitness plan:

1. Consult with a healthcare professional: It is critical to consult with your healthcare team before beginning or changing an exercise plan.

They can offer advice based on your specific health needs and assist you in understanding any precautions or modifications required for diabetes management.

2. Establish your objectives: Consider your workout objectives, such as controlling blood sugar levels, decreasing weight, enhancing cardiovascular health, or increasing general fitness. Setting clear goals will help you structure your routine more efficiently.

3. Select the appropriate exercises: Include a variety of aerobic, strength training, and flexibility exercises. Aerobic workouts such as brisk walking, cycling, swimming, and dancing increase cardiovascular fitness and aid in weight loss. Weight lifting and resistance band activities increase muscle mass, improve insulin sensitivity, and promote improved blood sugar control. Stretching and yoga are examples of flexibility activities that improve the

range of motion and help to prevent injuries.

4. Make a plan: Aim for at least 150 minutes of moderate-intensity aerobic activity per week, spaced out across at least three days. Consider dividing sessions into smaller chunks of time, such as 30 minutes every day or 10 minutes at various points during the day. Aim for at least two times per week of strength training activities that target key muscle groups. Remember to schedule recovery days.

5. Warm-up and cool-down: Make warming up before exercise and cooling down afterward a priority. Light aerobic activities should be performed for 5-10 minutes to gradually boost heart rate and loosen muscles. Similarly, stretch for 5-10 minutes at the end of each workout to minimize muscular tightness and prevent injuries.

6. Check blood sugar levels: Check your blood sugar levels before, during, and after exercise to see how your

body reacts. Measure your levels more regularly at first, until you become acquainted with your body's reactions. Adjust your food intake or medicine as directed by your healthcare team.

7. Stay hydrated: To stay hydrated, drink plenty of water before, during, and after exercise. Dehydration can impair blood sugar regulation, so drink plenty of fluids.

8. Pay attention to your body: During exercise, pay attention to how your body

feels. Stop and inform your healthcare expert if you suffer any symptoms such as chest pain, dizziness, or excessive exhaustion.

9. Progressively Increase Intensity and Length: Begin with a manageable level of intensity and duration and progressively increase over time to avoid overexertion or injury.

Remember that consistency is essential in sticking to a fitness plan. Regular physical activity, combined with a healthy diet and proper diabetes treatment, can significantly improve blood sugar control and general health.

Aerobic vs Strength Training

Aerobic (cardiovascular) workouts and strength training (resistance exercises) are both important components of a well-rounded fitness regimen, with each providing unique benefits for people with diabetes. Combining these two types of exercise can improve blood glucose control, cardiovascular health, muscle strength, and overall well-being.

Here's how aerobic and strength training workouts compare:

Cardiovascular (Aerobic) Exercises: Aerobic workouts are activities that raise your heart rate and breathing rate, so improving your cardiovascular fitness. These workouts work for vast muscle groups and help the heart and lungs work more efficiently. Examples of common aerobic activities include:

1. Walking: Walking is a low-impact activity that is good for the majority of people. It

is simple to incorporate into regular habits.

2. Cycling: Cycling is a fantastic cardiovascular sport that is easy on the joints, whether done on a stationary bike or outside.

3. Swimming: Swimming is a low-impact sport that gives a full-body workout while being easy on the joints.

4. Dancing: Dancing is a wonderful method to get active and raise your heart rate.

5. Jogging/Running: For those with a greater level of fitness,

jogging or running can be beneficial cardio exercises.

Benefits of Aerobic Exercises:

1. Increased insulin sensitivity and glucose uptake into cells during and after exercise to improve blood glucose management.
2. Weight control is advantageous for people with Type 2 diabetes or those attempting to maintain a healthy weight.
3. Lowering blood pressure, improving cholesterol levels, and lowering the risk of heart

disease all contribute to improved cardiovascular health.

4. Exercise causes the release of endorphins, which reduces stress and improves mood.

Strength Training (Resistance Exercises): Resistance exercises entail working against a resistance to grow and strengthen muscles. Body weight, resistance bands, free weights, or weight machines can all be used for this. Strength training exercises include the following:

1. Squats: These work the lower body, specifically the thighs, hips, and glutes.
2. Lunges: Lunges target the lower body's quadriceps, hamstrings, and glutes.
3. Push-ups: Push-ups typically work the chest, shoulders, and triceps.
4. Bicep Curls: These workouts work the biceps, which are located in the upper arms.
5. Planks: These exercises serve to develop the core muscles, which include the abdominals and back.

Diabetes Strength Training Advantages:

1. Increases muscular mass, which can boost metabolism and aid in weight loss.
2. Better blood glucose management due to increased insulin sensitivity.
3. Improves bone health and reduces the risk of osteoporosis.
4. Improved functional strength and balance, lowering the risk of falls and injuries.

Combining Aerobic and Strength Training: Combining aerobic and strength training routines can bring numerous benefits to diabetics. Aerobic workouts increase cardiovascular fitness and blood glucose control, whereas strength training helps grow and maintain muscle mass, which supports general metabolic health. Before beginning a new workout plan, always consult with your healthcare physician or a competent fitness trainer, especially if you have any existing health conditions or diabetic concerns.

Managing Blood Glucose During Exercise

Managing blood glucose during exercise is critical for diabetics to guarantee safety and maximize performance. Depending on factors such as intensity, duration, and type of activity, as well as individual responses to exercise, exercise can have varying impacts on blood glucose levels. Here are some tips for controlling blood glucose levels when exercising:

1. Determine Blood Glucose Levels: Check your blood glucose levels before

beginning any activity session. It may be unsafe to exercise if your blood glucose levels are too low (below 70 mg/dL or 3.9 mmol/L) or too high (over 250 mg/dL or 13.9 mmol/L with ketones). Before you begin your workout, address any abnormal blood glucose levels.

2. Exercise Timing: Think about when you exercise in relation to your meals and insulin doses. Exercise after meals may help reduce hypoglycemia in people with

Type 1 diabetes because eating provides a continuous source of glucose during activity. If you use insulin, you should be aware of how different forms of insulin may affect blood glucose levels during exercise. Rapid-acting insulin may produce hypoglycemia during or immediately after exercise, although long-acting insulin may not.

3. Adjust Insulin and Medications: Consult your healthcare practitioner if insulin dosages or diabetic

medications need to be adjusted for activity. Reduced insulin doses before or during exercise can aid in the prevention of hypoglycemia. To avoid blood glucose variations, this should be done under the supervision of a healthcare practitioner.

4. Choose the Right Snacks: If your blood glucose levels are lower than the ideal range before exercise, have a modest snack containing carbohydrates and protein around 30 minutes before

beginning your workout. This can aid in the prevention of hypoglycemia during physical activity.

5. Stay Hydrated: To stay hydrated, drink plenty of water before, during, and after exercise. Dehydration can influence blood glucose levels and cause other health problems.

6. Check Blood Glucose Levels During Exercise: Check your blood glucose levels on a regular basis throughout longer or more intensive activities, especially if you

are prone to hypoglycemia. During the activity, keep a blood glucose monitor and suitable snacks or glucose pills on hand.

7. Be Prepared for Hypoglycemia: If you suffer hypoglycemia symptoms (such as shakiness, dizziness, or confusion) while exercising, stop immediately and treat the low blood sugar with fast-acting carbohydrates such as glucose tablets or fruit juice.

8. Post-Exercise Monitoring: Continue to check your blood

glucose levels after exercise, since some people may have delayed hypoglycemia, several hours following physical activity.

9. Increase Intensity and Length Gradually: If you're new to exercise or haven't been active in a while, begin with lower-intensity exercises and gradually increase the intensity and length. This helps your body adapt to exercise and reduces the danger of blood glucose fluctuations.

10.   Pay Attention to Your Body: Pay attention to how your body reacts to various types of exercise and alter your regimen as necessary. Because everyone's body reacts differently to physical activity, it's critical to be aware of your own.

Blood glucose control during exercise necessitates careful planning, monitoring, and personalized changes. Develop a specific fitness plan with your healthcare provider or a certified diabetes educator that meets your needs and helps you maintain healthy blood glucose levels during physical activity.

Overcoming Barriers to Physical Activity

Overcoming physical activity hurdles is critical for diabetics to build a consistent exercise regimen and receive the many advantages of regular physical activity. Various difficulties can make staying active difficult, but with determination and some practical strategies, these obstacles can be efficiently tackled. Here are some frequent physical activity hurdles and solutions:

1. Inadequate Time:
   Solution: Break up your physical exercise into shorter, more manageable sessions to include it in your regular routine. use a 10-minute stroll during your lunch break, for example, or use the stairs instead of the elevator. Finding tiny chunks of time throughout the day might build up to the suggested amount of exercise.

2. Lack of Motivation:
   Set specific and attainable goals for your fitness regimen. Make a schedule or enlist the assistance of an exercise companion to hold you accountable and motivated. Make exercise a positive and fun experience by choosing activities that you enjoy.

3. Hypoglycemia Fear:
   Solution: Examine your blood glucose levels before and after exercise to see how your body reacts. To avoid hypoglycemia, schedule your

workouts after meals or have a little snack with carbohydrates and protein before you go. Carry fast-acting glucose sources, such as glucose tablets or fruit juice, with you throughout workouts in case your blood sugar drops.

4. Injury Fear:
Solution: Begin with low-impact exercises that are appropriate for your fitness level. As you gain confidence, gradually advance to higher-intensity workouts. To lessen the

chance of injury, warm up before each workout and include stretching exercises.

5. Environmental and Weather Factors: Solution: Maintain flexibility in your exercise regimen and have backup plans for indoor activities in case of inclement weather. Consider joining a club or fitness center that provides a wide range of indoor training possibilities.

6. Lack of Support: Seek help from friends, family, or support groups to keep you motivated and

encouraged on your fitness quest. Make exercising a social activity by doing it with a friend or family member.

7. Physical limits:
Solution: Consult with a healthcare physician or a trained fitness trainer who is familiar with diabetes management to build an exercise routine that takes into account your physical limits and health demands. Adaptive exercises and adjustments are provided to

accommodate a wide range of abilities.

8. Financial Restriction: Solution: Exercise does not have to be costly. Investigate free or low-cost activities such as walking, running, hiking, or using internet workout videos.

9. Lack of Information: Solution: Learn about the benefits of diabetes exercise and how to exercise properly. For advice on appropriate workouts for your condition, speak with a licensed fitness trainer or diabetes educator.

10.   Overcoming Mental Difficulties:
Solution: Identify and resolve any mental barriers or negative exercise beliefs. Use positive self-talk and concentrate on the benefits of physical activity, such as enhanced well-being and diabetes management.

Remember that incorporating physical activity into your daily routine may necessitate perseverance and adaptability. Begin cautiously, make realistic goals, and be gentle with yourself.

You can build an effective and pleasurable exercise regimen that contributes to improved blood glucose control and overall health by taking tiny measures to overcome impediments.

CHAPTER FIVE
Medications Options

Diabetes medication alternatives differ depending on the type of diabetes and the individual's health needs. There are three major classifications of diabetes: type 1 diabetes, type 2 diabetes, and gestational diabetes. Here's a rundown of the various drug alternatives for each type:

Diabetes Type 1:

Type 1 diabetes is a disease in which the body's immune system assaults and destroys beta cells in the pancreas responsible for the production of insulin. Individuals with Type 1 diabetes require insulin therapy to adequately maintain their blood glucose levels.

1) Insulin Injections: Most persons with Type 1 diabetes require numerous daily insulin injections or use an insulin pump to constantly supply insulin.

2) Insulin Types: Insulin comes in a variety of durations of action, including rapid-acting, short-acting, intermediate-acting, and long-acting insulin. The insulin regimen is customized to the individual's lifestyle and blood glucose control requirements.

Type 2 diabetes:

Type 2 diabetes is distinguished by insulin resistance and insufficient insulin production. Treatment options for Type 2 diabetes include lifestyle changes, oral medicines, and (if necessary) insulin therapy.

1) Lifestyle adjustments: For moderate cases of Type 2 diabetes, lifestyle adjustments such as eating a nutritious diet, increasing physical exercise, and keeping a healthy weight may be enough to effectively manage blood glucose levels.

2) Oral Medications:

- Metformin: Metformin is the standard first-line treatment for Type 2 diabetes. Metformin enhances insulin sensitivity by decreasing hepatic glucose production.

- Sulfonylureas: These drugs cause the pancreas to produce more insulin.
- DPP-4 Inhibitors: These medications assist control blood glucose levels by preventing the breakdown of incretin hormones, which boost insulin release while suppressing glucagon secretion.

- GLP-1 Receptor Agonists: GLP-1 receptor agonists operate similarly to incretin hormones, boosting insulin secretion, decreasing glucagon secretion, and slowing stomach emptying.
- SGLT-2 Inhibitors: These drugs prevent glucose reabsorption in the kidneys, resulting in increased urine glucose excretion.

3) Insulin Therapy: When oral drugs fail to manage blood

glucose levels, or if diabetes worsens, insulin therapy may be added to the treatment regimen.

Gestational Diabetes:

Gestational diabetes occurs during pregnancy and is usually manageable via lifestyle changes such as a balanced diet and regular physical activity. To regulate blood glucose levels during pregnancy, insulin therapy or oral medicines may be used in some circumstances.

Individuals with diabetes must collaborate closely with their healthcare professionals to develop the best pharmaceutical regimen for them based on their specific type of diabetes, overall health state, blood glucose control goals, and personal preferences.

Medication management is only one part of diabetes treatment, and it is frequently used in conjunction with lifestyle changes to achieve optimal diabetes management and general well-being.

Insulin Therapy: Types, Delivery Methods and Administration

Insulin therapy is an essential component of diabetes management, particularly for those with Type 1 diabetes and in certain situations, Type 2 diabetes. Insulin therapy works by replacing or increasing the body's natural insulin to assist regulate blood glucose levels. An overview of insulin kinds, delivery techniques, and administration is provided below:

I.   Types of Insulin:

Insulin is categorized into numerous categories based on its onset, peak, and duration of activity. The most common insulin kinds are:

- Rapid-Acting Insulin: It begins functioning 15 minutes after injection, peaks in 1 to 2 hours and lasts 3 to 4 hours. Insulin lispro, insulin aspart, and insulin glulisine are a few examples. Rapid-acting insulin is frequently used to cover meals and lower blood glucose levels.

- Short-Acting (Regular) Insulin: It begins to work within 30 minutes to an hour, peaks in 2 to 3 hours, and lasts 4 to 6 hours. During specified instances, regular insulin is routinely used to cover meals or control blood glucose levels.

- Intermediate-Acting Insulin: It begins to operate in 2 to 4 hours, peaks in 4 to 12 hours, and lasts 12 to 18 hours. NPH insulin is one example. Background insulin coverage between meals and nighttime is frequently provided by intermediate-acting insulin.

- Long-Acting Insulin: It has a long onset of action and delivers insulin in a constant stream with no discernible peak. Insulin glargine, insulin detemir, and insulin degludec are a few examples. Long-acting insulin is used throughout the day and night to provide basal insulin coverage.

II.   Delivery Methods:

Insulin can be provided in a variety of ways, the choice depending on individual preferences and lifestyle:

- Insulin Injections: Subcutaneous injections using insulin pens or syringes are the most prevalent route of insulin delivery. Insulin pens are pre-filled with insulin and offer a handy method of measuring and administering insulin doses. Syringes are widely used to draw insulin from vials and allow for more precise dosage.

- Insulin Pumps: These are small devices that continually supply rapid-acting insulin through a tiny catheter implanted beneath the skin.

They give a consistent basal insulin rate while also allowing for bolus injections to cover meals or correct elevated blood glucose levels. Insulin pumps provide flexibility and may be chosen by some people due to their ease of use.

III.   Insulin Administration:

Adequate insulin administration is critical for maintaining adequate blood glucose control and lowering the risk of complications. Here are some general insulin administration guidelines:

- Injection Sites Should Be Rotated: To prevent lipodystrophy (changes in the fat tissue under the skin) and to guarantee continuous insulin absorption, rotate injection sites within the same injection location (e.g., belly, thighs, upper arms) on a regular basis.

- Injection Timing: Follow your healthcare provider's guidelines for insulin injection timing and frequency. Rapid-acting insulin is usually given just before or after meals, whereas long-acting insulin is usually given once or twice a day.
- Injection Technique: Clean the injection site with an alcohol swab, squeeze the skin (if necessary) to form a small fold, and enter the

needle at a 90-degree angle (or as indicated by your healthcare practitioner).

- Dose Modification: Collaborate with your healthcare physician to change insulin doses depending on blood glucose monitoring, activity level, and dietary consumption.
- Insulin should be stored correctly: To keep insulin effective, follow the storage instructions. Insulin should be kept in the refrigerator and kept away from severe heat.

Always seek individualized insulin therapy and administration advice from your healthcare practitioner or a certified diabetes educator. Proper insulin control, in conjunction with lifestyle changes and regular blood glucose monitoring, is critical for efficient diabetes management and general health.

Oral Medications for Diabetes

Individuals with Type 2 diabetes are frequently offered oral diabetes medicines to assist regulate blood glucose levels. These drugs improve insulin sensitivity, reduce glucose synthesis by the liver, and increase insulin secretion in diverse ways. It's vital to remember that oral drugs aren't used to treat Type 1 diabetes because the condition necessitates insulin therapy. The following are the primary types of oral diabetic medications:

1. Metformin: Metformin is the first-line drug for Type 2 diabetes and is frequently administered in conjunction with lifestyle changes. It is a biguanide drug that reduces

glucose synthesis in the liver while boosting insulin sensitivity in peripheral tissues. Metformin does not induce weight gain and may possibly result in a minor weight decrease.

2. Sulfonylureas: Sulfonylureas cause the pancreas to produce more insulin. They are available in several generations, each with a distinct duration and dose frequency. Glipizide, glyburide, and glimepiride are examples of sulfonylureas. These drugs

can help lower blood glucose levels, but they can also cause hypoglycemia (low blood sugar), especially if taken in excess or if meals are omitted.

3. DPP-4 Inhibitors: DPP-4 inhibitors act by preventing the breakdown of incretin hormones, which promote insulin release and reduce glucagon secretion. DPP-4 inhibitors assist reduce blood glucose levels by extending the activity of these hormones. Sitagliptin, saxagliptin, linagliptin, and

alogliptin are a few
examples.

4. GLP-1 Receptor Agonists
(Glucagon-like Peptide-1
Receptor Agonists): GLP-1
receptor agonists mimic the
action of incretin hormones,
increasing insulin secretion
while decreasing glucagon
secretion and slowing
stomach emptying. These
drugs are accessible as
injectables (rather than pills)
and can aid in weight loss.
Exenatide, liraglutide,
dulaglutide, and semaglutide
are a few examples.

5. SGLT-2 Inhibitors (Sodium-Glucose Cotransporter-2 Inhibitors): SGLT-2 inhibitors operate by preventing glucose reabsorption in the kidneys, which results in increased urine glucose excretion. This method lowers blood glucose levels and may have further benefits for heart and renal health. Empagliflozin, canagliflozin, dapagliflozin, and ertugliflozin are a few examples.

6. Thiazolidinediones (TZDs): TZDs increase insulin

sensitivity in peripheral tissues. They are used less frequently due to potential negative effects such as weight gain and an increased risk of heart failure. Pioglitazone and rosiglitazone are types of TZDs.

7. Alpha-Glucosidase Inhibitors: Alpha-glucosidase inhibitors prevent carbs from being absorbed in the digestive tract, leading to a slower rise in blood glucose levels after meals. Alpha-

glucosidase inhibitors include acarbose and miglitol.

It's crucial to remember that the choice of oral medication(s) will be influenced by a number of factors, including the individual's blood glucose control, overall health, the existence of other medical disorders, and any medications used to treat other health issues.

Always follow your healthcare provider's medication recommendations and talk to them about any issues or questions you have about your diabetes treatment plan. Furthermore, combining oral drugs with lifestyle changes such as eating a balanced diet and exercising regularly helps improve diabetes management and general well-being.

Non-Insulin Injectable Medications

Non-insulin injectable medicines are a class of drugs used to control blood glucose levels in people with Type 2 diabetes. These drugs are given via injection; however, they are not insulin. They lower blood glucose levels, improve insulin action, and decrease glucose synthesis in the liver via multiple processes. The following are the primary types of non-insulin injectable medications:

1. GLP-1 Agonists (Glucagon-like Peptide-1 Receptor Agonists): GLP-1 receptor agonists are injectable drugs that replicate the activity of the incretin hormone GLP-1, which occurs naturally in the body. These drugs increase insulin secretion, decrease glucagon secretion (which decreases glucose synthesis

in the liver), and slow stomach emptying. Examples are:

- Exenatide (Byetta, Bydureon)
- Liraglutide (Victoza, Saxenda)
- Dulaglutide (Trulicity)
- Semaglutide (Ozempic, Rybelsus)

2. Amylin Analogs: Amylin is a hormone that is co-secreted with insulin by pancreatic beta cells. It aids in blood glucose regulation by slowing stomach emptying

and decreasing glucagon output. Amylin analogs are injectable medicines that work similarly to amylin. They work in conjunction with insulin or oral medicines to improve blood glucose management, especially after meals. Pramlintide (Symlin) is the only approved amylin analog.

3. SGLT-2 Inhibitors (Sodium-Glucose Cotransporter-2 Inhibitors): While most SGLT-2 inhibitors are taken orally, there is one injectable medicine in this family that is

given once a week. SGLT-2 inhibitors prevent glucose reabsorption in the kidneys, resulting in increased urine glucose excretion. SGLT-2 inhibitors assist reduce blood glucose levels by eliminating excess glucose from the body via urine. The injectable SGLT-2 inhibitor is known as: Semaglutide (Ozempic) - A once-weekly injectable version is available.

These non-insulin injectable drugs offer an additional treatment option for persons with

Type 2 diabetes who may experience difficulties with oral medications or require extra glucose-lowering agents to meet their blood glucose targets. It's vital to remember that the type of injectable drug chosen will be determined by personal criteria such as blood glucose management, overall health, and treatment goals.

It is critical, as with any diabetic treatment, to follow your healthcare provider's advice regarding the use of non-insulin injectable drugs. Regular blood glucose monitoring and constant communication with your healthcare team can assist ensure that your diabetes management strategy is effective and safe. Furthermore, lifestyle changes such as eating a nutritious diet and engaging in regular physical activity can supplement the effects of medication and help to better diabetes management and general well-being.

Combination Therapies
Combination therapy for diabetes entails the use of numerous drugs with distinct mechanisms of

action in order to improve blood glucose control. These techniques are often utilized for Type 2 diabetes patients who may not attain their goal blood glucose levels with a single prescription or who require additional glucose-lowering medications to successfully control their illness. Oral medicines, non-insulin injectables, and/or insulin can all be used in combination therapy. Here are some popular ways to combination therapy:

1. Combination of Oral Drugs: Different classes of oral

drugs can be combined to treat different elements of glucose management. Metformin, for example, can be taken with sulfonylurea or a DPP-4 inhibitor. Metformin can be used in conjunction with a GLP-1 receptor agonist. A DPP-4 inhibitor with an SGLT-2 inhibitor can be coupled.

2. Conjunction of Injectable drugs: Non-insulin injectable drugs can also be used in conjunction. GLP-1 receptor agonists, for example, can be used with SGLT-2 inhibitors.

GLP-1 receptor agonists can be used with insulin.

3. Insulin Combinations: Different forms of insulin can be mixed to give both basal (background) and prandial (mealtime) insulin coverage for people with Type 2 diabetes who require insulin therapy. Before meals, a common insulin combination is basal insulin (long-acting) mixed with rapid-acting insulin. Basal insulin is paired with GLP-1 receptor agonists to provide basal and postprandial coverage.

4. Triple Therapy: Some people may require more complete blood glucose management, which may necessitate the use of triple therapy. Typically, triple therapy consists of an oral medicine (e.g., metformin), a GLP-1 receptor agonist, and an SGLT-2 inhibitor. This method may be especially effective for people who are unable to control their symptoms with oral drugs alone. The individual's blood glucose control, overall health, treatment goals, and

reaction to previous drugs will all influence the decision of combination therapy. Always consult with your healthcare professional to find the best combination therapy for your diabetes control.

CHAPTER SIX

Diabetes Complications and Risk Management

Diabetes is a complex and chronic disease that, if not well treated, can lead to a variety of complications. Controlling blood glucose, blood pressure, and cholesterol levels, as well as living a healthy lifestyle, are critical in lowering the risk of problems. Here are some frequent diabetic complications:

1. Cardiovascular Complications
2. Diabetic Retinopathy (Eye Complications)
3. Diabetic Neuropathy (Nerve Damage)
4. Diabetic Nephropathy (Kidney Damage)
5. Hypoglycemia etc.

Cardiovascular Complications

Cardiovascular problems are a major issue for diabetics and one of the most prevalent and dangerous long-term health hazards linked with the illness. Diabetes can have a significant impact on the cardiovascular system, raising the risk of developing a variety of cardiovascular diseases. Diabetes is related to two major cardiovascular complications:

1. Coronary Artery Disease (CAD): Coronary artery disease occurs when the blood channels that carry oxygen and nutrients to the heart muscle (coronary arteries) narrow or become clogged by a buildup of fatty deposits known as plaques. Diabetes is a major risk

factor for the onset of CAD. When CAD worsens, it can cause chest discomfort (angina), heart attacks (myocardial infarction), and other problems.

2. Stroke and Peripheral Artery Disease (PAD): Diabetes raises the risk of having a stroke and developing peripheral artery disease. A stroke happens when blood arteries in the brain get blocked or rupture, resulting in decreased blood flow and potential brain damage. Peripheral artery disease

affects the blood vessels outside the heart, most commonly in the legs, and can result in pain, decreased mobility, and, in extreme cases, gangrene and amputation.

Diabetes Risk Factors for Cardiovascular Complications:

Several factors contribute to diabetes patients' higher risk of cardiovascular problems, including:

1. Poor Blood Glucose Control: High blood glucose levels can damage blood vessels

and raise the risk of atherosclerosis (hardening and constriction of arteries) over time.

2. High Blood Pressure: Diabetes can result in high blood pressure (hypertension).

3. High Cholesterol Levels

4. Obesity

5. Smoking

6. Physical Inactivity

Nerve Damage and Neuropathy

Diabetic nerve injury, often known as neuropathy, is a common and devastating consequence. Elevated blood glucose levels can cause nerve damage throughout the body, most typically affecting the extremities, such as the feet and hands, over time. Neuropathy can cause a variety of symptoms and problems, ranging from minor discomfort to substantial impairment. Diabetic neuropathy can be classified into numerous kinds, including:

1. Neuropathy of the Periphery: The most frequent type of diabetic neuropathy is peripheral neuropathy, which affects the peripheral nerves, which convey messages between the brain, spinal cord, and the rest of the body. It usually affects the feet and legs, although it can also affect the hands and arms.

   Symptoms could include:
   - Tingling or burning sensation
   - Numbness or sensitivity to touch

- Sharp, piercing pains
- Muscle fatigue
- Balance and coordination problems

Peripheral neuropathy can cause foot sores and infections, which, if left untreated, can lead to significant problems such as gangrene and amputation.

2. Neuropathy of the Autonomic Nervous System: The autonomic nerve system, which controls involuntary bodily activities such as heart rate, blood pressure, digestion, and

bladder function, is affected by autonomic neuropathy. Symptoms could include:

- Heart rate or blood pressure fluctuations
- Gastroparesis (slow stomach emptying) and other digestive issues
- Bladder issues, such as incontinence or retention
- Sexual impotence
- Sweating dysfunction

If not treated effectively, autonomic neuropathy can lead to serious problems such as cardiac rhythm issues and gastrointestinal complications.

3. Proximal Neuropathy (Radiculoplexus Neuropathy): Nerves in the thighs, hips, buttocks, or legs are affected by proximal neuropathy. It can result in significant discomfort, muscle weakness, and trouble moving, most commonly on one side of the body. Proximal neuropathy is more likely in people over the age of 65 who have Type 2 diabetes.

4. Focal Neuropathy: Focal neuropathy occurs when a single nerve or a small group of nerves is damaged, resulting in immediate, acute, and localized pain. It can affect any nerve in the body and usually happens unexpectedly.
Symptoms are:
- Intense discomfort in the head (cranial neuropathy)
- Torso or leg pain (focal neuropathy in the trunk or limb)

- Eye vision difficulties (focal neuropathy)
- Bell's palsy (paralysis of the facial nerve)

Prevention and Management

Maintaining blood glucose levels within the desired range is critical for preventing and slowing the course of neuropathy.

1. Medical Check-ups on a Regular Basis: Regular screenings and monitoring by healthcare practitioners are critical for early detection and intervention.

2. Foot Care: Individuals with peripheral neuropathy must take care of their feet. Inspecting feet for injuries or changes on a regular basis, wearing suitable footwear, and keeping feet clean and dry can all assist to avoid issues.

Adopting a healthy lifestyle, which includes a balanced diet, frequent physical activity, quitting smoking, and managing stress, can improve general well-being and help manage neuropathy symptoms.

Kidney Disease and Diabetes Nephropathy

When it comes to diabetes, kidney disease, also known as diabetic nephropathy, is a common and significant consequence that can develop. Diabetic nephropathy is a kind of kidney disease characterized by damage to the kidney's tiny blood arteries, resulting in reduced kidney function and an increased risk of kidney failure. It is a leading cause of end-stage renal disease (ESRD), which requires dialysis or kidney transplantation.

Although the actual origin of diabetic nephropathy is unknown, it is closely connected to prolonged periods of increased blood glucose levels. Chronic high blood glucose levels can harm the blood vessels of the kidneys, impairing their ability to filter waste and excess fluids from the blood.

Other variables that can lead to diabetic nephropathy include:

- Diabetes for a long time with poor blood glucose control
- Hypertension (high blood pressure)

- Predisposition due to genetics
- Smoking
- Kidney illness runs in the family.

Diabetic Nephropathy Stages:

- Stage 1 (Microalbuminuria): The kidneys begin to leak little amounts of protein (albumin) into the urine in the early stages. This is detectable with a simple urine test.
- Stage 2 (Macroalbuminuria or Proteinuria): As kidney disease progresses, more protein is secreted in the

urine, indicating more severe kidney impairment.

- Stage 3 (Nephropathy): The kidneys' ability to filter waste materials and fluids deteriorates further, resulting in kidney function reduction.
- Stage 4 (Advanced Nephropathy): Kidney function declines further, and problems such as fluid retention, anemia, and electrolyte abnormalities may occur.
- Stage 5 (End-Stage Kidney Failure): Kidney function is substantially reduced at this

point, and the kidneys are unable to sustain life. Dialysis or kidney transplantation may be required at this stage.

Prevention and Management

Preventing or postponing diabetic nephropathy requires comprehensive diabetes care as well as preventive kidney health measures:

1. Blood Glucose Control: It is critical to keep blood glucose levels within the desired range in order to reduce the risk of kidney injury.

2. Blood Pressure Control: It is critical to keep blood pressure at a healthy level in order to protect the kidneys. Even if blood pressure is not markedly raised, medications to decrease blood pressure, such as ACE inhibitors or ARBs, are frequently administered to diabetics.

3. Regular Medical Exams: Regular kidney function screenings, which include urine and blood tests (e.g., serum creatinine and estimated glomerular filtration rate), are critical for

early identification and intervention.

4. Medication Management: In addition to blood pressure drugs, healthcare providers may prescribe medications to control additional risk factors.

5. Lifestyle Modifications: Adopting a healthy lifestyle is critical in the prevention and management of kidney disease. Among the lifestyle strategies is a healthy diet that is low in salt and saturated fat can help lessen

the strain on the kidneys and blood vessels.

6. Physical Activity: Getting enough exercise on a regular basis can enhance overall health and help control blood glucose and blood pressure levels.

7. Smoking is harmful to renal function and cardiovascular health. Quitting smoking is critical for lowering the risk of renal disease.

Eye Complications and Diabetes Retinopathy

Diabetes patients are concerned about eye issues, notably diabetic retinopathy. Diabetes retinopathy is a disorder that causes damage to the blood vessels in the retina, which is the light-sensitive tissue at the back of the eye. It is the major cause of vision loss and blindness in diabetic individuals. The two types of diabetic retinopathy are:

1. Diabetic Retinopathy Without Proliferation (NPDR): The blood vessels in the retina weaken and leak in the early stages of diabetic retinopathy, known as NPDR, resulting in the formation of microscopic bulges known as microaneurysms. As the situation worsens, the blood vessel walls may become blocked, resulting in insufficient blood supply to the retina.

2. Diabetic Retinopathy (PDR): In the more advanced stage, a

lack of adequate blood supply to the retina causes the formation of new, aberrant blood vessels. These delicate veins are prone to bleeding, which can result in scar tissue formation, retinal detachment, and significant vision loss.

Diabetic Retinopathy Risk Factors:

Several factors contribute to the development of diabetic retinopathy.

1. Diabetes Duration: The longer a person has diabetes,

the greater the chance of getting retinopathy.

2. Blood Glucose Control: Uncontrolled blood glucose levels raise the risk of ocular problems.

3. Management of Blood Pressure: High blood pressure can aggravate retinopathy and raise the risk of visual loss.

4. Diabetic nephropathy (kidney illness) is linked to an increased risk of diabetic retinopathy.

Prevention and Management

1. Eye Exams on a Regular Basis: Early identification and intervention are critical in preventing vision loss. Diabetes patients should have complete dilated eye exams at least once a year.
2. Blood Pressure Control: It is critical to keep blood pressure at a healthy level in order to protect the blood vessels in the eyes.
3. Changes in Lifestyle: Adopting a healthy lifestyle that includes a well-balanced

diet, frequent physical activity, not smoking, and stress management can help with general well-being and eye health.

4. Diabetic Retinopathy Treatment: Diabetic retinopathy treatment is dependent on the severity of the condition. Among the treatment options available are:

5. Photocoagulation (Laser Therapy): Laser therapy is used to seal leaking blood vessels and slow the

formation of aberrant blood vessels.

6. Anti-VEGF (vascular endothelial growth factor) drugs may be injected into the eye to minimize edema and prevent the formation of new blood vessels.

7. Vitrectomy surgery may be performed in advanced cases of diabetic retinopathy with extensive hemorrhage or retinal detachment to remove the vitreous gel and scar tissue from the eye.

8. Regular communication with healthcare providers and eye

experts, as well as adherence to medical advice and continuing monitoring of blood glucose levels and eye health, are critical for preserving vision and preventing diabetic retinopathy-related consequences.

Foot Care and Amputation Prevention

Foot care is an important part of diabetes management, especially for people who have peripheral neuropathy or impaired circulation. Proper foot care can help prevent issues like foot ulcers and infections, as well as lower the chance of amputation. Diabetes patients should adhere to the following foot care guidelines:

1. Check your feet every day for cuts, blisters, redness, swelling, or changes in skin color or warmth. If you can't see the bottom of your feet, use a mirror or contact a family member for assistance.

2. Maintain Clean and Dry Feet: Wash your feet regularly with warm water and a little

soap. To avoid fungal infections, gently pat them dry, especially between the toes. Soaking your feet may result in maceration of the skin.

3. Moisturize: Use a moisturizer to keep the skin on the tops and bottoms of your feet moistened and avoid dryness and cracking. To avoid excessive moisture retention, avoid putting moisturizer between the toes.

4. Trim Toenails Carefully: Use a nail file to smooth the edges of your toenails and

trim them straight across. To prevent ingrown toenails, avoid cutting into the corners or cutting them too short.

5. Proper Footwear: Wear shoes that are comfortable and allow enough room for your toes to move. Look for shoes that are breathable and give support and cushioning. High heels and open-toed shoes should be avoided.

6. Socks: Put on clean, dry socks that fit properly and do not bunch up. To keep your feet dry, wear socks made of moisture-wicking fabrics.

7. Do not smoke: Smoking lowers blood flow and can affect foot circulation, increasing the risk of foot issues.

8. Regular Foot Exams: Have your feet checked by a healthcare practitioner at regular check-ups or as directed by your doctor. Inform your healthcare physician if you detect any foot problems.

9. Protect Feet from Extreme Temperatures: Avoid going barefoot on hot surfaces, and in cold weather, wear thick

socks and insulated, waterproof shoes.

10.   Be Active: Exercise on a regular basis to improve circulation and overall health.

11.   Avoid Self-Treatment: If you discover any foot problems, don't try to treat them on your own. Seek medical help as soon as possible from a healthcare practitioner or a foot expert (podiatrist).

Amputation Avoidance:

Taking proactive steps to care for your feet can greatly lower the chance of amputation in diabetics. To further avoid amputation, it is critical to:

1. Control Foot Ulcers Promptly: If you get a foot ulcer, seek medical assistance right once. Prompt treatment can help to avoid infection and other problems.
2. Follow the advice of your healthcare provider: Follow your healthcare team's treatment plans and recommendations, including wound care instructions and medication management.

3. Attend regular foot examinations: Consult a podiatrist or foot expert on a regular basis to evaluate your foot health, especially if you have a history of foot issues or neuropathy.

4. Continue Your Education: Discover the importance of regular foot care and diabetes treatment. Attend diabetes education classes to stay up to date on how to prevent foot issues.

CHAPTER SEVEN

Emotional Well-Being and Diabetes

The term "emotional well-being" refers to a person's total mental and emotional health. It includes sentiments of happiness, contentment, and life satisfaction, as well as the ability to cope with stress, control emotions, and maintain positive relationships. When it comes to diabetes, mental well-being is critical in managing the condition. Diabetes is a chronic illness that necessitates daily self-care, such as blood sugar monitoring, medication administration, and healthy lifestyle choices. Diabetes can be difficult to manage and can have a substantial influence on a person's mental and emotional health. Diabetes patients frequently confront the following emotional challenges:

1. Stress: Diabetes management can be stressful since it demands constant focus and vigilance to keep blood sugar

levels within the target range.
Stress can impair blood sugar
management and make it
difficult to manage the
disease.

2. Anxiety and Depression:
   Studies reveal that people
   with diabetes have a higher
   chance of getting anxiety and
   depression than those who do
   not have the condition.
   Constant concern about blood
   sugar levels, potential
   complications, and the
   impact of diabetes on daily
   life can all contribute to
   mental health problems.

3. Diabetes Distress: Diabetes distress is a type of emotional load associated with the difficulties of living with diabetes. Feelings of irritation, exhaustion, and being overwhelmed by the obligations and expectations of diabetes control are all part of it.

4. Body Image Issues: Diabetes can sometimes cause changes in body weight, looks, or physical ability, which can have an impact on a person's body image and self-esteem. This can lead to feelings of

uneasiness, humiliation, or dissatisfaction with one's physical appearance.

5. Social and Emotional Support: Living with diabetes may necessitate lifestyle modifications that have an impact on one's social life. Emotional distress can be exacerbated by feelings of isolation or a lack of support from family, friends, or healthcare experts.

Individuals with diabetes must address their emotional well-being in order to properly manage their condition and maintain a high quality of life. Here are some ways for improving emotional well-being:

1. Seek Support: Join a diabetes support group, talk to family and friends, or consult with a diabetes-specific mental health expert. Sharing your feelings and experiences with those who understand can be a source of comfort and support.
2. Develop Healthy Coping Mechanisms: Create healthy coping methods to deal with

stress and tough emotions. Engage in regular physical activity, also practice relaxation techniques (such as deep breathing or meditation), or discover interesting hobbies and pastimes.

3. Communicate with Healthcare Providers: It is critical to communicate with healthcare providers about any emotional issues or concerns associated with diabetes in an open and honest manner. They can offer advice, resources, and

assistance to help you manage your emotional well-being.

4. Self-Care: Prioritize self-care activities that enhance general well-being, such as obtaining adequate sleep, eating nutritious food, and engaging in enjoyable and relaxing activities.

5. Education and Knowledge: Educate yourself on diabetes self-care and management options. Understanding the disease and its implications can help alleviate worry and

empower you to take charge of your health.

6. Create a Supportive Environment: Surround yourself with people who understand and support your diabetes management efforts. Family, friends, healthcare practitioners, and diabetic support organizations are all examples of people who can help.

Taking care of one's emotional well-being is an important aspect of effectively controlling diabetes. Individuals with diabetes can enhance their overall quality of life and manage the demands of their condition by addressing emotional challenges.

Coping with the Emotional Impact of Diabetes

Diabetes can be difficult not just physically, but also emotionally. Coping with the emotional effects of diabetes is critical for overall health. The following are some useful strategies:

1. Recognize and acknowledge your emotions: Recognize and acknowledge your sentiments concerning

diabetes. It is common to experience a variety of emotions such as annoyance, rage, grief, or fear. Accepting these feelings is a necessary step toward learning how to control them.

2. Educate yourself: Find out everything you can about diabetes. Understanding the disease, its management, and treatment alternatives can help you feel more empowered and less anxious. Consult with healthcare specialists, read credible resources, join support

groups, or attend diabetes education events.

3. Seek support from family, friends, or support groups: Seeking assistance from family, friends, or support groups can help you feel understood and less alone with your diabetes. Share your thoughts, worries, and victories with people who can relate to your path. Finding a diabetes group can bring a sense of belonging and encouragement.

4. Practice self-care: It is critical to take care of your

emotional well-being. Find activities that bring you joy and relaxation, such as hobbies, mindfulness practice, spending time in nature, or listening to music. Make time for yourself and emphasize self-care to prevent diabetes-related stress and anxiety.

5. Seek professional assistance: If you are feeling overwhelmed by your emotions or trying to cope with the effects of diabetes, consider obtaining professional assistance. A

therapist or counselor can help you manage the emotional issues that come with living with diabetes.

6. Set attainable objectives: Setting attainable goals for diabetes management might help you feel more in control and minimize stress. Divide larger ambitions into smaller, more manageable tasks. Celebrate each step along the journey, and be gentle with yourself if you encounter difficulties.

7. Engage in healthy coping skills, such as frequent

exercise, practicing relaxation techniques (e.g., deep breathing, meditation, yoga), writing, or indulging in artistic endeavors. These hobbies can help you relax and feel better emotionally.

8. Communicate with your healthcare team: Keep open and honest lines of communication open with your healthcare team. Discuss any diabetes-related problems or difficulties you are experiencing. They can offer advice, support, and

help with any physical or mental concerns that emerge.

9. Maintain a positive mindset: Concentrate on the positive aspects of your life and enjoy your accomplishments. Surround yourself with positive people and take inspiration from those who have successfully managed their diabetes. Recognize and appreciate your efforts in managing the disease, even if the outcomes aren't always ideal.

10.   Stay informed: Stay current on the newest developments in diabetes management. New diabetes-management technologies, therapies, and services are continually being developed. Being well-informed might help you feel more empowered and hopeful about your diabetes journey.

Remember that dealing with the emotional consequences of diabetes is an ongoing journey. Be gentle with yourself and seek help when necessary. You can build successful techniques for navigating the emotional problems that come with living with diabetes with time and practice.

Building a Support Network
Individuals dealing with diabetes must establish a support network. A solid support system can offer emotional encouragement, practical aid, and useful resources to assist in effectively managing the challenges of diabetes. Below are some guidelines for creating a supporting network:

1. Family and Friends: Begin by contacting close family members and friends. Share your diabetes journey with them, educate them on the disease, and explain how they can help you manage your diabetes. It can be really reassuring to have loved ones who understand and are there for you.

2. Diabetes Support Groups: Join a diabetes support group in your area or online. These groups are made up of people who understand the specific challenges of living

with diabetes. Participating in these organizations can provide you with a sense of belonging as well as opportunities to share your experiences and learn from others.

3. Healthcare Team: Members of your healthcare team, such as doctors, diabetes educators, and dietitians, are critical members of your support network. Establish open communication with them, share your problems, and seek advice on how to

effectively manage your diabetes.

4. Online Communities and Forums: Diabetes support can be found on a variety of online platforms and forums. Participating in these groups can connect you with people all around the world who have had similar experiences and can offer practical guidance and emotional support.

5. Diabetes Education Programs: Attend diabetes education classes or seminars. These programs

give useful diabetes management knowledge and can assist you in developing the necessary skills for living well with the illness.

6. Mental Health Professionals: If you are experiencing major emotional distress or mental health issues as a result of your diabetes, consider seeking help from a mental health expert who is familiar with diabetes care.

7. Diabetes Organizations: Get in touch with diabetes organizations like the American Diabetes

Association or Diabetes UK, which provide a variety of resources, activities, and support networks for those living with diabetes.

8. Support at Work or School: Inform your company or school about your diabetes and any accommodations you may require. When your colleagues, professors, or classmates are aware of your condition, they can offer understanding and support.

9. Social Media: On social media, follow diabetes influencers and advocates.

Engaging with these people can provide a sense of community as well as access to diabetes-related information.

10.   Recreational or Hobby Groups: Get involved with clubs or groups that are relevant to your interests or hobbies. Activities that you enjoy can help relieve stress and give you a good outlet for diabetes-related feelings.

Stress Management Techniques

Stress management is essential for diabetes treatment because it can alter blood sugar levels and general health. Here are some techniques for managing stress:

1. Exercise: Regular physical activity can help lower stress levels. During exercise, we release endorphins which are natural mood boosters. Include activities that you enjoy in your schedule, such as walking, swimming, dancing, or yoga.
2. Relaxation techniques: Use relaxation techniques such as deep breathing, meditation, guided visualization, or

progressive muscle relaxation. These methods can help you calm your mind, reduce stress, and encourage relaxation.

3. Time management: To avoid feeling overwhelmed, organize and prioritize your responsibilities. Make a timetable or to-do list to help you manage your time and minimize unneeded stress. If possible, delegate work and learn to say no when required.

4. Maintain a healthy lifestyle by eating well-balanced

food, getting enough rest, and staying hydrated. These behaviors can benefit your general well-being and provide a solid foundation for stress management.

5. Support network: Seek assistance from family, friends, or support groups. Talking to someone who understands your circumstance might provide emotional support and comfort. Consider attending diabetes support groups to connect with people who

may be going through similar experiences.

6. Stress-relieving activities: Engage in relaxing and unwinding activities such as reading, listening to music, having a warm bath, practicing a hobby, or spending time in nature. Discover hobbies and activities that make you happy and make out time for them.

7. Practice mindfulness: Mindfulness entails being totally present at the moment and observing your thoughts

and feelings without judgment. It can help alleviate tension and induce relaxation. Consider incorporating mindfulness meditation into your daily activities, such as eating or walking.

8. Get organized: Keeping track of your diabetes supplies, prescriptions, and appointments will help to reduce stress. To keep on schedule and feel more in charge of your diabetes management, use tools such

as calendars, reminders, or smartphone applications.

9. Seek professional assistance: If stress becomes overwhelming and begins to interfere with your everyday life, consider obtaining professional assistance. A therapist or counselor can offer advice and assistance in dealing with diabetes-related stress.

10.   Reduce stress or exposure: Identify and reduce sources of stress in your life. Setting boundaries, avoiding triggers, and

making essential lifestyle changes are all possible. Recognize that you have power over how you respond to stressors and make decisions that put your well-being first.

Remember that stress management is a constant practice. Understand that it might take time to figure out what techniques are suitable for you. Be kind to yourself and open to exploring new ways. You may create effective stress management practices that work for you and support your goals with constant practice.

Setting Goals and Finding Motivation

Setting objectives and finding motivation is critical for optimal diabetes management. Here are some pointers to help you develop and maintain goals:

1. Create SMART goals: SMART goals- Specific, Measurable, Achievable, Relevant, and Time-bound goals. Instead of a broad objective like "improve blood sugar control," set a precise

target like "reduce my HbA1c levels by 0.5% in the next three months by following my meal plan and exercising for 30 minutes five times a week."

2. Break it down: If your goals seem daunting, divide them into smaller, more doable tasks. This makes them less intimidating and helps you to more easily track your progress. To keep motivated, celebrate each small accomplishment along the road.

3. Determine your why: Determine why diabetes management is important to you. What long-term benefits do you hope to achieve? This could include bettering your general health, avoiding issues, or maintaining a great quality of life. Remembering your why can help you stay motivated even when faced with obstacles.

4. Educate yourself: Learn about the benefits of successful diabetes management as well as the consequences of failing to

keep your condition under control. Understanding the consequences of your choices can be a strong incentive. To stay inspired and educated, keep up with the newest research and breakthroughs in diabetes care.

5. Seek help: Surround yourself with a caring network of family, friends, or a diabetes support group. Share your goals with them and solicit their support and responsibility. When you have someone to share your path with, you can get

motivation and support when you need it.

6. Track your progress: Using a notebook, smartphone app, or diabetes management software, keep track of your blood sugar levels, medication or insulin intake, exercise regimen, and other pertinent aspects. Visualizing your progress can be motivational and useful for staying on track.

7. Reward yourself: Reward yourself on a regular basis for meeting your goals. It could be doing something you

enjoy, taking a day off, or doing something you enjoy. This type of positive reinforcement can keep you motivated and provide something to look forward to.

8. Visualize success: Visualize yourself successfully controlling your diabetes and reaching your objectives. Consider the good results and how they will affect your life. This mental image can motivate you and boost your confidence in your talents.

9. Maintain a good attitude and focus on your success rather

than obsessing over setbacks. Every step forward, no matter how tiny, should be celebrated. Surround yourself with positive people and look for inspiring stories or role models who have successfully managed diabetes. To stay motivated, use positive affirmations and self-talk to strengthen your commitment.

10.   Be open to adapting and revising your goals as you proceed through your diabetes management journey. Your requirements

and circumstances may vary over time, so you should reassess and adapt your goals accordingly. This adaptability will assist you in remaining motivated and going forward.

Maintaining a Positive Outlook
Individuals dealing with diabetes must have a good attitude. Here are some techniques for cultivating a good mindset:

1. Educate yourself: Learn about diabetes, how it is managed, and the most recent advances in therapy. Knowledge enables you to

make informed judgments, which can boost your confidence while decreasing emotions of doubt.

2. Concentrate on what you can control: Recognize that you cannot control every aspect of diabetes. Instead, concentrate on things you can control, such as your daily habits, nutrition, exercise routine, and medication adherence. You can restore control and positivity by channeling your energies toward doable objectives.

3. Seek help: Seek the help of family, friends, or those who understand your diabetes journey. Connect with diabetes support groups or online communities to share experiences, get insights, and be encouraged.

4. Recognize and appreciate accomplishments: Recognize and celebrate your accomplishments, no matter how minor they may appear. Give yourself credit for your efforts and progress, whether it's improving your blood sugar control, attaining a

health-related milestone, or implementing beneficial lifestyle adjustments.

5. Engage in self-care activities: Participate in activities that encourage self-care and well-being. Regular exercise, mindfulness or meditation, pursuing hobbies, spending time with loved ones, and prioritizing self-care activities that offer you joy and relaxation are examples of such activities.

6. Use positive self-talk: Pay attention to your internal dialogue and fight negative

thoughts or self-criticisms. Replace negative thoughts with positive affirmations and reminders of your diabetes management strengths and efforts.

7. Set achievable and realistic goals for yourself: Set achievable and realistic goals for yourself. Divide them into smaller, more doable steps. Celebrate each milestone you achieve because it will drive you to keep going.

8. Seek professional assistance: If you are having difficulty maintaining a happy attitude

or dealing with emotional issues associated with diabetes, consider seeking professional assistance from a therapist or counselor. They can offer advice and support in regulating your emotions and keeping a positive attitude.

CHAPTER EIGHT

Living with Diabetes: Practical Tips and Strategies

Diabetes necessitates daily management and lifestyle changes. Here are some helpful hints and ideas for navigating life with diabetes:

1. Build a diabetes management plan with your healthcare team: Work with your healthcare team to build a personalized diabetes

management strategy.
Monitoring your blood sugar
levels, taking prescribed
medications, following a
healthy food plan, engaging
in regular physical activity,
and arranging regular check-
ups may all be part of this
approach.

2. Check your blood sugar
levels on a regular basis with
a glucose meter, as directed
by your healthcare
professional. Keeping track
of your levels might help you
discover patterns and make

required lifestyle or treatment plan changes.

3. Adopt a healthy eating plan: Eat a well-balanced diet rich in nutrient-dense foods. Choose whole grains, lean proteins, fruits and vegetables, and healthy fats instead. Consume fewer sugary drinks, processed foods, and high-sodium meals. Consider consulting with a licensed dietitian who specializes in diabetes to assist you in developing a specific meal plan.

4. Participate in regular physical activity: Include regular exercise in your routine. As directed by your healthcare physician, aim for at least 150 minutes of moderate aerobic activity or 75 minutes of vigorous-intensity aerobic activity every week. Physical activity can aid in the reduction of blood sugar levels, the improvement of insulin sensitivity, and the maintenance of a healthy weight.

5. Take medications as directed: If your doctor has recommended medications to help you control your diabetes, be sure you take them. To keep blood sugar levels stable, stick to the prescribed dosage and schedule.

6. Diabetes education: Learn about diabetes management, treatment options, potential consequences, and how to avoid or manage them. Attend instructional programs, read credible resources, and keep up with

the newest research to be informed.

7. Manage stress: Because stress can affect your blood sugar levels, find healthy strategies to cope with it. Pursue activities that you enjoy and that will help you relax. Seek emotional stress management assistance from family, friends, or support groups.

8. Make sleep a priority: Aim for 7-9 hours of quality sleep per night. Sleep deprivation can have an impact on blood sugar regulation and general

health. Create a consistent sleep schedule, a bedtime routine that promotes relaxation, and a comfortable sleeping environment.

9. Stay hydrated: Drink enough water throughout the day to stay hydrated. Water promotes healthy overall health and proper physiological functions.

10.   Communicate with your healthcare team as follows: Maintain open and honest communication with your medical staff. Schedule appointments on a regular

basis to review your diabetes care, ask questions, and address any problems or challenges you may be experiencing. This partnership can assist you in staying on track with your treatment plan and making any necessary adjustments.

11.   Prepare for emergencies by stocking a diabetes emergency pack with necessary supplies such as glucose tablets or gel, insulin, syringes, and a glucagon emergency kit. Carry a medical identification card,

and notify your loved ones and close contacts about your diabetes and what to do in an emergency.

12.   Seek help: Contact family, friends, or support groups for emotional support and understanding. Joining a diabetes support group can provide you with a sense of community while also allowing you to learn from others who are living with diabetes.

Traveling With Diabetes

Traveling with diabetes necessitates additional planning and preparation to ensure that you can manage your health efficiently while away from home. Here are some helpful hints and ideas to make your travels more fun and safer:

1. Consult Your Medical Team: Make an appointment with your healthcare physician to discuss your travel plans before you leave. They can assist you in assessing your health status, adjusting

prescriptions as needed, and providing important travel information.

2. Bring Extra Supplies: Bring enough diabetes supplies, such as insulin, oral pills, test strips, lancets, and glucose monitoring devices. It is preferable to over-pack than to run out of important products during your trip.

3. Keep diabetic prescriptions and Supplies in Your Carry-On: Instead of checking your diabetic prescriptions and supplies, pack them in your carry-on bag. This keeps

them conveniently available during the journey and eliminates the danger of losing them if your checked luggage is lost.

4. Travel Insurance: Think about getting travel insurance that covers pre-existing medical issues, such as diabetes. This insurance can safeguard you financially in the event of an unexpected medical emergency during your trip.

5. Prescriptions and Medical Information: Carry a letter from your healthcare

physician outlining your diabetes treatment plan, medications, and any medical equipment required. Ensure to have a list of emergency contacts, including your doctor's phone number.

6. Be Aware of Time Zone Changes: If you're traveling across time zones, consult with your healthcare team about adjusting your insulin levels and prescription schedules.

7. Stay Hydrated and Mindful of Meals: Drink plenty of water throughout your

journey to stay hydrated. Even while traveling, be careful of your meals and snacks and strive to keep a balanced diet.

8. Maintain Regular Blood Glucose Monitoring: Maintain regular blood glucose monitoring, especially if your travel routine includes changes in physical activity and eating patterns.

9. Be Prepared for Security Checks: Inform airport or other travel checkpoint security staff about your

diabetic supplies. To assist with security screenings, pack your prescriptions and equipment in clear, labeled bags.

10.   Prepare for Hypoglycemia: Keep fast-acting glucose sources on hand, such as glucose pills or gels, to treat hypoglycemia episodes as soon as they occur. In case of low blood sugar, always keep snacks or carbohydrates on hand.

11.   Maintain Physical Activity While Traveling: Try to incorporate physical

activity into your vacation, such as taking brief walks during layovers or stretching during long flights or vehicle journeys.

12. Adjust Mealtime Insulin dosages: If your travel schedule affects your meal timings, consult with your healthcare team about adjusting your mealtime insulin dosages.

13. Exercise Caution with Food and Water: When visiting new places, exercise caution with food and water. Stick to well-cooked, hot

meals and, if required, bottled water.

14.   Inform Travel Companions: Inform your travel companions about your diabetes and how they can assist you in the event of a medical emergency.

15.   Prepare for Emergencies: Learn about the local emergency services and medical facilities at your destination.

Remember that planning and preparation are essential for a successful diabetic journey.

Sick Day Management

Diabetes management during sick days demands extra attention and care. Here are some sick-day management tips:

1. Check blood sugar levels more frequently than normal: Check your blood sugar levels more regularly than usual. Illness can impact blood sugar levels, so it's critical to stay alert and respond appropriately.

2. Stay hydrated: To stay hydrated, drink plenty of fluids, particularly water.

Staying hydrated can help prevent dehydration, which is prevalent during illness and can have an impact on blood sugar levels.

3. Keep taking diabetic prescriptions: Unless otherwise directed by your healthcare practitioner, keep taking your diabetes medications, including insulin, even if you are eating less or are unable to eat. Keeping your blood sugar levels constant throughout illness is critical.

4. Eat regular meals if possible: Try to stick to your regular meal schedule, but if you can't, eat small, frequent meals or snacks that incorporate carbohydrates and protein. If you have a poor appetite, focus on foods that are easy to digest, such as soups or broths.

5. Modify insulin dosages as needed: If your healthcare professional instructs you, modify your insulin dosages based on your blood sugar levels and any particular sick day instructions. Working

with your healthcare team to determine the proper changes for your individual circumstance is critical.

6. Treat symptoms: If you have symptoms such as fever, nausea, or vomiting, follow your healthcare provider's advice on how to treat them. Over-the-counter drugs should be used with caution because some may contain components that can influence blood sugar levels.

7. Consult your healthcare provider: If you have serious symptoms or your blood

sugar levels are regularly high or low, consult your healthcare provider. They can give you personalized guidance depending on your specific needs.

8. Rest and stress management: Give your body the rest it requires to recuperate. Because stress can alter blood sugar levels, it's critical to keep stress levels as low as possible during illness.

9. Inform others: Tell your loved ones, close contacts, and coworkers about your

diabetes and what to do in an emergency. If necessary, they can offer aid and support.

10.   Implement a Sick Day Emergency Plan: Work with your healthcare provider to develop a Sick Day Emergency Plan. This plan provides guidelines for managing your diabetes while you're sick, such as when to contact your healthcare provider, what to do if you can't eat, and how to alter medications or insulin dosages.

Managing Diabetes at Work or School

Living with diabetes while juggling work or school duties can be a unique challenge. However, by employing effective tactics and prioritizing self-care, it is feasible to successfully navigate this circumstance. Individuals with diabetes can effectively control their condition in these environments by taking proactive actions. To develop understanding and support, it is critical to raise awareness and educate others about diabetes. Open communication with supervisors, instructors, or teachers is essential for discussing unique diabetic concerns and accommodations. Planning meals and snacks ahead of time aids in maintaining stable blood sugar levels. Blood glucose levels are monitored on a regular basis to maintain proper management. Physical activity and exercise play an important part in diabetes control and should be included in everyday activities.

Stress management is also essential, as stress can alter blood sugar levels. It is critical to carry vital supplies and medication, such as insulin and glucose monitoring devices, in order to be prepared for any eventuality. Finally, taking regular breaks to attend to diabetes-related requirements is essential for general well-being.

Living with diabetes at work or school might be difficult, but it is possible to successfully manage the illness. Raising diabetes awareness and educating others is critical for building a supportive environment. It is critical to communicate openly with supervisors, teachers, or professors about special needs and adjustments. Planning meals and snacks ahead of time helps to keep blood sugar levels stable.

Regular blood glucose monitoring is essential for optimal control. Exercise and physical activity should be incorporated into everyday activities to help with diabetes management. Stress management is critical since stress can affect blood sugar levels. It is critical to keep required supplies and medication, such as insulin and glucose monitoring devices, on hand at all times. Finally, taking regular breaks to address diabetes-related needs is critical for general health.

Tips for Socialising and Dining Out

Individuals with diabetes may face specific obstacles when socializing and dining out. You may, however, enjoy these adventures while efficiently managing your diabetes with some planning and mindfulness. Here are some pointers to assist you handle social gatherings and eating out:

1. Plan Ahead: If you know you'll be dining out or attending a social function, make sure your meals and snacks are prepared correctly. If possible, look over the menu ahead of time to make healthier choices.

2. Select Restaurants Wisely: Choose eateries that provide a variety of healthy options, such as salads, grilled proteins, and veggies.

3. Portion Control: Watch your portion amounts, especially while eating high-carb items. Consider sharing large

servings or requesting a to-go container to conserve leftovers.

4. Modify Your Order: Do not be afraid to request changes to your meal, such as replacing starchy sides with more veggies or serving dressing on the side.

5. Limit Sugary Beverages: Instead of sugary drinks, choose water, sparkling water, or unsweetened beverages. Consume alcohol in moderation and avoid sugary cocktails.

6. Avoid Mindless Snacking: It's tempting to graze on appetizers and snacks at social gatherings. Keep an eye on your intake and choose healthy selections wherever possible.

7. Be Wary of Hidden Sugars: Many sauces, dressings, and condiments contain hidden sugars. To limit your intake, request these things on the side.

8. Check Your Blood Glucose: If you're trying new meals or are unsure how they'll affect your blood glucose, test

before and after your meal to see how they affect you.

9. Bring Snacks: Bring a few nutritious snacks with you when you go out to avoid harmful temptations and low blood sugar.

10.   Communicate Your Needs: Don't be afraid to tell your friends or dining partners about your diabetes control requirements. They will most likely understand and support you.

11.   Stay Active: Include physical activity in your daily routine, including on social

occasions. After a meal, go for a walk or indulge in a physical activity that you enjoy.

12. Mindful Eating: Savor each bite, chew gently, and pay attention to hunger and fullness signs to practice mindful eating.

13. Eat Dessert in Moderation: If you desire dessert, share it with others or choose a smaller piece.

14. Drink Water Throughout the Event: Drink water throughout the event to stay

hydrated and avoid confusing thirst with appetite.

15.   Recognize Progress: Recognize your abilities to navigate social gatherings and dining out while effectively controlling your diabetes. Recognize and praise yourself when you make healthy decisions.

Remember that managing diabetes in social situations is all about finding a happy medium between having fun and putting your health first. With time and practice, you'll grow more at ease socializing and dining out while controlling your diabetes.

Pregnancy and Gestational Diabetes

Pregnancy is a joyful and exciting time, but it can also bring with it some additional health concerns, such as gestational diabetes. Gestational diabetes is a kind of diabetes that develops during pregnancy and normally goes away once the baby is born. Proper gestational diabetes care is critical for a safe pregnancy and delivery. Here are some important strategies to consider:

1. Regular Monitoring: In order to manage gestational diabetes, blood sugar levels must be monitored on a regular basis. This aids in the detection of blood sugar variations or irregularities, allowing for early adjustments in diet, exercise, or medication if necessary.

2. Healthy and Balanced Diet: A healthy and balanced eating plan is essential for managing gestational diabetes. Consuming a range of nutrient-dense foods such as fruits, vegetables, whole

grains, lean meats, and healthy fats is normal. It is critical to limit your intake of sugary meals and beverages.

3. Physical Activity: As directed by your healthcare physician, frequent physical activity can help control blood sugar levels. Walking, swimming, and prenatal yoga can all be useful. However, before beginning or continuing any fitness routine during pregnancy, talk with your healthcare physician.

4. Medication and Insulin: In some circumstances, lifestyle changes may not be enough to regulate blood sugar levels in women with gestational diabetes. To assist control your disease, your doctor may prescribe medicine or insulin injections. It is critical to heed their advice and directions carefully.

5. Prenatal Care: It is critical to have regular prenatal check-ups and appointments during pregnancy, especially if you have gestational diabetes.

Your healthcare professional will monitor your blood sugar levels, evaluate your overall health, and give you any required guidance and assistance.

6. Blood Sugar Monitoring at Home: In addition to frequent clinic visits, your healthcare practitioner may urge you to use a glucose meter to check your blood sugar levels at home. This allows you to monitor your levels throughout the day and make any required

dietary or prescription changes.

7. Education and Support: Attending diabetes education programs or support groups designed exclusively for pregnant women can provide vital knowledge, resources, and emotional support. It can help you understand your illness better and connect with people who are going through similar things.

8. Postpartum Screening: It is critical to have postpartum screening to monitor blood sugar levels after giving

birth. This assists in determining if gestational diabetes has resolved or if more therapy or monitoring is required.

Remember that women with gestational diabetes can have a good pregnancy and delivery with careful management.

CONCLUSION: Empowering Your Diabetes Journey

To summarize, living with diabetes might be difficult, but it does not define who you are or limit your potential. Taking ownership of your health, embracing self-care, and making informed decisions to live a full life is all part of empowering your diabetes journey. We've covered many different areas of understanding and controlling diabetes in this detailed guide.

We've covered the essential foundations of diabetes treatment, from delving into the complexities of diabetes kinds and causes to the importance of blood glucose monitoring, insulin therapy, and medication alternatives. We've also discussed the significance of nutrition and food management, highlighting the relevance of carbohydrates, proteins, and lipids in keeping a healthy macronutrient balance.

We've also talked about the effects of sugars and artificial sweeteners, mindful eating, and stress management techniques, emphasizing the importance of emotional well-being in diabetes care. We've looked at how exercise and physical activity can help with diabetes management and provided advice on how to create tailored exercise regimens.

We've also talked about how to manage diabetes complications and the necessity of risk management. Foot care, eye issues, and kidney illness have all been investigated, emphasizing the significance of preventive care and early intervention.

Aside from the medical components, we've recognized the need of developing a strong support network, finding encouragement from loved ones, and maintaining a happy attitude throughout your diabetes journey.

The guide has provided practical methods to handle different environments while properly managing diabetes, whether you're at work, school, or socializing with friends. We've also talked about the specific challenges of pregnancy and gestational diabetes, emphasizing the importance of prenatal care and monitoring.

Diabetes empowerment entails education, resilience, and advocacy. You may take control of your health and well-being by being informed, obtaining support from healthcare professionals and loved ones, and maintaining a positive attitude.

Remember that every step you take to improve your diabetes management is a step toward a healthier, more happy life. Accept opportunities for development and learning, and appreciate your accomplishments, no matter how minor. Your diabetes path is unique to you, and with dedication and self-compassion, you can thrive and live a life defined by your strength and resilience rather than diabetes.